BEAUTIFUL EYES
THE ULTIMATE EYE MAKEUP GUIDE

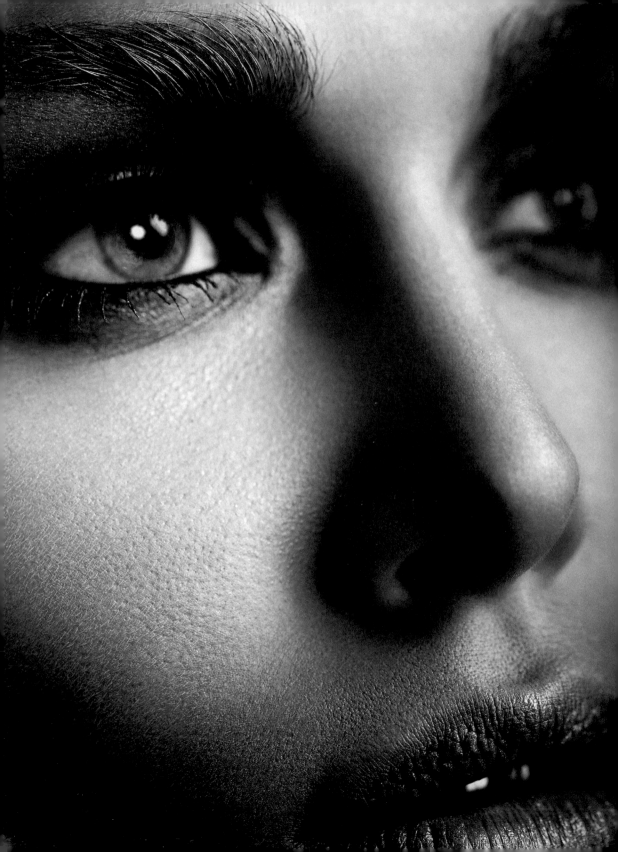

RAE MORRIS
BEAUTIFUL EYES
THE ULTIMATE EYE MAKEUP GUIDE

Photography by Steven Chee

ARENA
ALLEN&UNWIN

First published in 2009

Arena Books, an imprint of
Allen & Unwin
83 Alexander Street
Crows Nest NSW 2065
Australia

Phone: (61 2) 8425 0100
Fax: (61 2) 9906 2218
Email: info@allenandunwin.com
Web: www.allenandunwin.com

Cataloguing-in-Publication entry is available
from the National Library of Australia
www.librariesaustralia.nla.gov.au

ISBN 978 1 7423 7087 3

Design: Seymour Designs

Printed in China at Everbest Printing Co

10 9 8 7 6 5 4 3 2

contents

MODEL: CATHERINE MCNEIL - CHIC MODELS • HAIR: MICHAEL BRENNAN - THE ARTIST GROUP

introduction

I fell into makeup. Well, not literally, although I have done that too. What I mean is makeup crept up on me and took me by surprise. I started my working life as a hairdresser, and it was in this guise that I found myself at the Miss Model of the World pageant in Istanbul in 1993. There I was, quietly at work on a model's hair, little knowing that destiny, in the shapely form of Naomi Campbell, was about to rear its extremely beautiful head.

Naomi was on the other side of the room with a male makeup artist when, suddenly, there was a flurry of angry voices then he was heading for the door in a flood of tears. In the stunned silence that followed, Naomi glared around the room and fortunately (although it didn't feel that way at the time) her gaze fell on me. 'Fix my lips,' she said. I looked at her mouth, then at the lip gloss on the bench, then back to her mouth. A wave of completely unwarranted confidence swept over me and I thought, 'How hard can it be?'

Before I had the chance to talk myself out of it, I picked up the lip gloss and got to work with only moderately shaky hands. As I did, the door burst open and the whole room erupted in a blaze of flashlights. The paparazzi had arrived … Next thing I knew, my picture was plastered all over the tabloids and my makeup career had officially begun. So before I go on, I'd like to say a belated thanks to Naomi for the dummy spit that made all this possible.

Fast-forward fifteen years and I now find myself writing a book. And I suppose the important question is, 'What makes this book any different from all the others that are out there?' Well, first of all, this book is designed to bring high-end fashion makeup into the realm of everyday life and into the hands of the everyday consumer. Every single look (even the most glamorous one) has a simple step-by-step photo guide and clear, concise instructions to help even the most inexperienced beginner apply the makeup.

Another thing I've aimed to do is to teach you makeup in exactly the same way that I do it and teach my assistants and students. I've included all the simple, practical tips, time-saving measures and shortcuts (or cheats, if you like) that I employ on a daily basis, to achieve those amazing results you see in magazines. So not only have I tried and tested them all, I've made them super-easy to follow.

Remember, just like any technique, makeup requires practice. If you don't get it right the first time round, don't stress. I have been doing it for years and I still have to wipe it all off and start again from time to time. So pick up your brushes, your lipsticks and your blushes and practise, practise, practise. And don't forget to have fun with it!

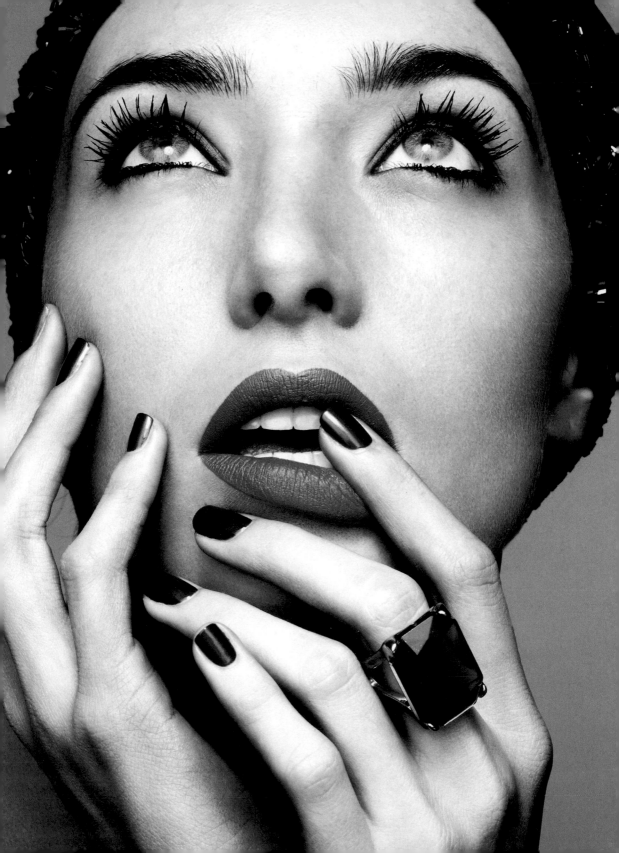

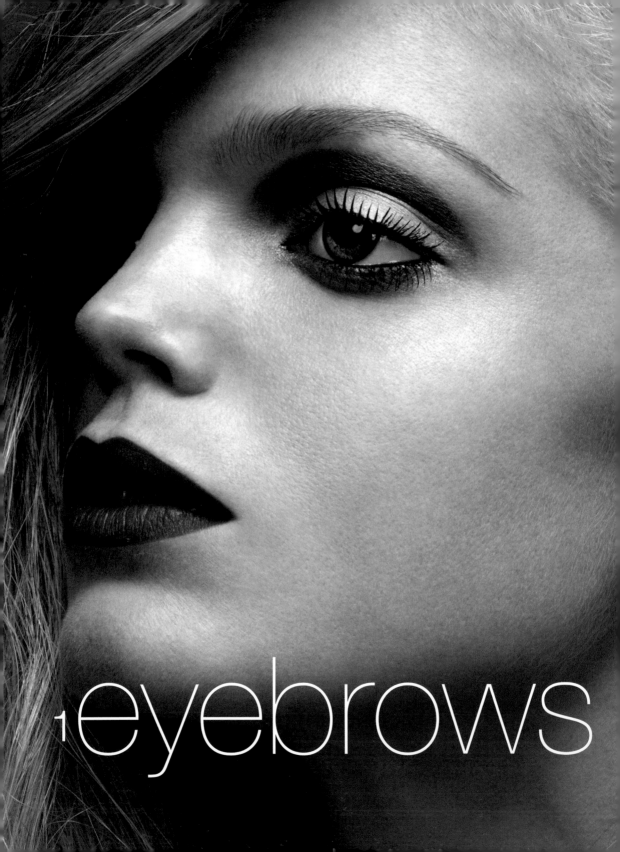

1eyebrows

When it comes to facial features, little has more power and impact than the shape of your brows. Get the shape right and you have an instant face-lift effect. Get it wrong and it can cause all sorts of problems. For instance, many women don't realise that their eyebrow shape can visually alter the look of their nose (for all the wrong reasons). What's more, the colour of your brows can either harden your features or take years off.

Great brows frame your eyes—they hold everything together and give your features definition and strength. As a makeup artist, when I'm shooting beauty for high-end fashion magazines, I always cast models based upon their brows.

If there is one section of this book I want you to take special notice of, it's this one. There's no point in doing glamorous or sexy eye makeup if you have eyebrows that look like caterpillars, slugs or tadpoles.

The number one 'crime' on my eyebrow offence list is over-plucked brows. Most women think that thin, highly arched brows lift the eye and make you look younger. However, they do the complete opposite. So let's start with the types of brows you should *not* have.

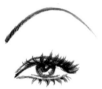

Type: Over-plucked. Hairs have been tweezed to oblivion, and there's barely a brow to be seen.
Effect: You've just aged yourself by ten years! Not to mention given yourself puffy-looking lids and a slight eye-droop.

Type: Tadpole brows, aka commas.
Effect: Extremely unattractive. These brows do nothing for you and the question on every makeup artist's lips is: 'Why? Who did this to you? And have you looked at a clown lately?'

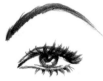

Type: The big 'M'. As in, semi-circle brows that look like they need a compass to navigate them.
Effect: First, these are the opposite of sophisticated (read: tarty). Second, they add five kilos instantly— this is the best way to add weight (in a bad way) to your face. Third, they make your nose look bigger. And fourth, they make your eyes look droopy.

Type: The downhill.
Effect: Speaks for itself. Just look closer at this sketch: sad, sad eyes; hello, puffy eyelids. These brows do nothing but make you look haggard and tired.

Type: The parting of the Red Sea.
Effect: Wide-set brows give you a blank expression and you look a little alien-ish. In terms of features, they throw the whole face out of balance, and they widen your nose like you would not believe.

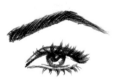

Type: The triangle.
Effect: These brows mean you're peaking too soon. By lifting the brow in the middle of the eye, you're causing a downhill puffy eyelid, and distorting your eye shape. It makes your eyebrows look like arrows pointing at the sky. This is a very hard look.

how to rehab your brows

If any of the above brows belong to you, then my advice is an urgent brow rehab! But if yours don't strictly fit in with these types of brows, how can you tell if your brows suit you? First, look at yourself closely in the mirror. Study your eyes and brows and then completely cover your brows with your index fingers. Look at your eyes again. Do they look better with or without your current brows? If the answer is 'without', this says that your brows are doing more harm than good to your look. Now, don't run for the wax pot! Book an appointment with a brow specialist (someone with good word-of-mouth reputation—ask your well-browed friends where they go), who will be able to design the perfect brow shape for you.

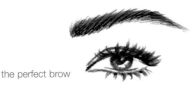

the perfect brow

How to achieve the perfect brows

Have you ever been told to start your eyebrows from an imaginary line upwards from your outer nostril or from the inner corner of your eye? In this scenario, if you have a wide nose or flared nostrils, you should start your brows closer to your eyeballs, with a huge gap in between. Right? Wrong!

As you can see from the following photos, a harsh arch in the wrong place can create a puffy eye and uneven brows are the right ingredients for a drooping or lopsided face. Likewise, a gap that is too big between a set of brows can actually make a nose look really big. That is why having the right brow shape is essential. The correct brow can make eyes look bigger, rectify unevenness, straighten your nose and make your face much more striking. In other words, the correct brow is important in making a beautiful face and therefore makeup.

The easiest way to achieve a foolproof brow is to follow a few small rules and three long lines.

1 Everyone has different-sized nostrils and noses, so your imaginary line must follow the natural line of the outer bridge of your nose. Got it? That is where your first brow hairs need to start! Then you can de-mono-brow all you like on the other side of this line.

2 Now, from that bridge line, draw another line that passes along the outer rim of your pupil and upwards. This is the highest point of any arch or height of the brow. This incline should smoothly follow the natural shape of your own brow. It's important to note that the arch isn't in the centre of the brow—it is very much off-centre, making the eye longer, sexier and with no 'surprised' look!

3 Finally, again, from the bridge line draw a line to the outer corner of your eye. This is where your brow should end.

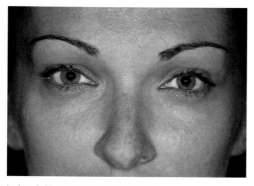
before (with over-plucked eyebrows)

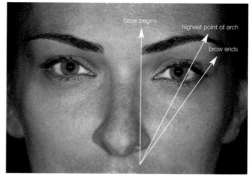
after (with the perfect eyebrows)

brow lightening

DO NOT TRY THIS AT HOME. Brow lightening must only be done by a fully qualified hairdresser because it's not as easy as it looks, and as you are working very close to the eye, you can cause some damage if you don't do it properly. You know how difficult it can be to colour the hair on your head; well, the same qualifications are needed to bleach brows (that's why hardly any makeup artists do it).

So why lighten? Because lightening the brows can be one of the most 'softening' techniques you can do. It's great when you change your hair colour—for example, if you go from being a blonde to a redhead, by colouring your brows a soft chestnut it makes your new hair colour look more natural, and it will soften your overall look. What's more, bleaching your brows has a softening effect on the hair itself, which is fantastic if you have brow hair like barbed wire.

If you want to lighten your brows but are a little scared about how they may end up looking, you can take a sneak preview by using brow mascaras (or hair mascaras—they were horrible on the hair to which they were supposed to add highlights, so due to bad sales they are hard to find, but they are fantastic on the brows). Just comb the colour mascara on and see what it looks like.

You can also darken your brows. As brow hairs fall out in cycles every six to eight weeks, any colour change is never permanent.

So to sum up, don't try it at home, and test brow-colour changes by using brow mascaras. And remember, it's only hair, and if you don't like it you can colour it back.

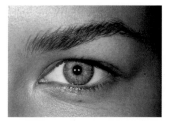
before lightening

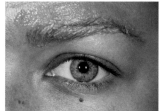
during lightening

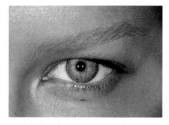
after lightening

brow tips

1   Your brows must suit you! If they don't, get them shaped by a professional.

2   Trim any extra-long hairs on your brows, but ideally, this would be done by your brow expert (even your hairdresser can come in handy for this one).

3   Always check brows from the side—use a second mirror to see your profile view.

4   Match your brow pencil to your brow hair colour, not your desired hair colour, as the difference would be too obvious.

5   If you lighten your hair colour on your head, then consider lightening your brows.

6   Buy brow mascaras—my favourite tool in this area. They are great for temporarily lightening or darkening the brow, as they have a gel formula which holds them into place. Brow mascara comes in many colours; if you're a redhead, you can buy one that matches your head hair colour, to tonally tie everything together.

7   Don't wax your brows on the day of an important event, because wax removes a light layer of skin and makes it impossible for foundation and eye shadow to adhere.

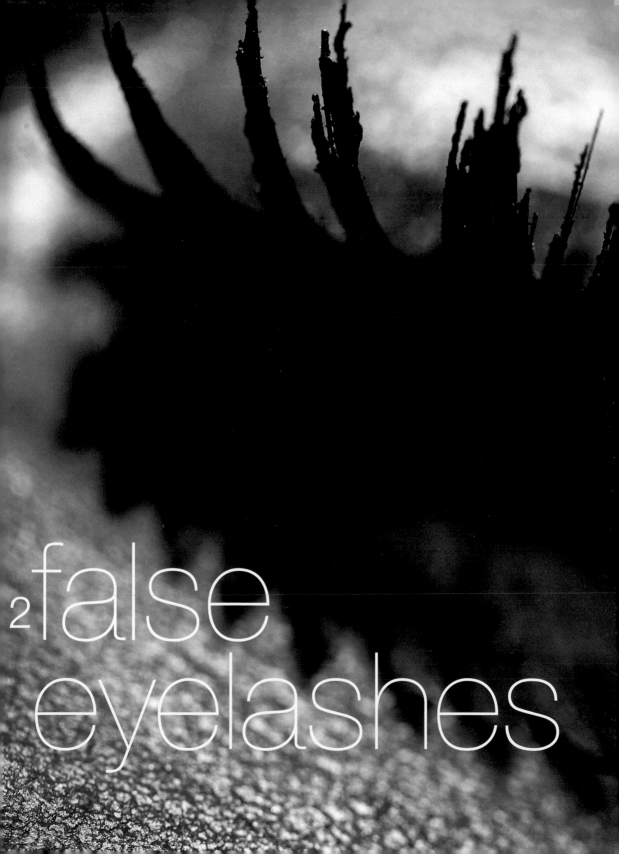

false
eyelashes

false lashes are like shoes—they either fit or they don't! If they don't fit correctly, they are uncomfortable, they can fall off or, worse, they will look fake when you don't want them to.

As a makeup artist, I use some sort of false lash in nearly every makeup I do. My two favourite things in makeup are mascara (as important as the air we breathe) and false lashes. If I don't have lashes in my kit, I go into a complete panic and I'll send assistants running for miles. I have even been caught cutting tiny hairs from models' heads (without them noticing) and sticking them on—now, that's desperation!

Most women don't realise that lashes, when applied by professionals, are measured to fit your exact lash line. This involves measuring the lash line and comparing it with the length of the false lash, and if it's too long or too short either the false lash has to be cut, or single lashes need to be added. You can do this yourself. Remember that 80 per cent of lashes will fit all eye shapes, but if the ones you buy are too long, then all you need to do is cut them.

I have found that in most cases a full lash is not required. For me, the sexiest look is when single lashes or just one-quarter is used on the outer lash line; this gives a winged effect and lifts the eyes instantly.

You can reuse false lashes (I don't because of hygiene). If you're using them for your eyes only, just soak them in warm water for 5 minutes to remove the glue before reusing.

As with anything there are do's and don'ts, so before you launch yourself into applying false lashes take note of the following.

Don't

- overuse glue, as it will not dry and can go into your eyes
- apply the lash if the glue is too wet; just squeeze a tiny amount onto the back of your hand and wait for it to get a little tacky, then apply it to the back of the false lash—not your lash line
- trim the false lash after you have applied it; you can cut your own lashes (I guarantee it!)—this is strictly for professionals only
- use lashes that are too heavy for your natural lashes to hold, as they drag your lash line down
- apply lashes too far out on your lash line if you have rounded eyes as they will drag your lash line down (see illustrations opposite).

Do

- curl your own lashes before applying falsies; if you attempt it afterwards, you can rip them off
- check the base of the lash; for example, if the lash (being a full lash) has a black line at its base, remember it will give you the look of an eyeliner, which you may or may not want
- paint the base after application if it is white (use liquid liner).

applying false eyelashes

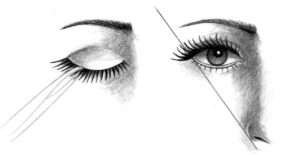

This illustration (above) clearly demonstrates how NOT to apply a false lash. As you can see, if you are looking down and apply the lash all the way to the end of your natural lash line, when you look up the false lash will drag down, causing the eye to droop. Also, it can cause a nasty shadow under the eye.

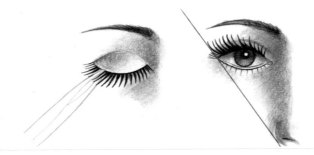

This is the correct way to apply false lashes. Notice that the lash has been moved inwards about half a centimetre. This ensures that when you look straight ahead, your lashes follow that beautiful line that gives your eyes a lift (from the corner of the nose to the corner of your eye). This instantly makes you look YOUNGER. The same applies with a single lash: always start approximately half a centimetre inwards. This rule rarely applies for Asian eyes because the eyelid is straighter and you don't have the issue of the lash drooping on the ends.

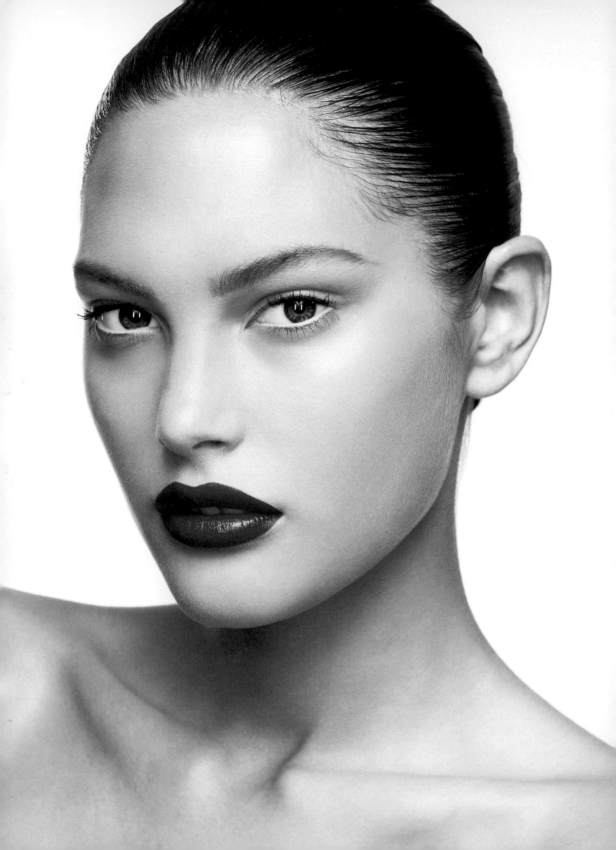

the power of lashes

I have used the next few pages to show you that false lashes have the power to dramatically change the way your eyes look. You can completely alter your eye makeup with just a lash. There are many different types of false lashes on the market. In fact, there are so many, no one would blame you for feeling confused and overwhelmed. So, over the next six pages, I show you three of the many possibilities you can achieve with false lashes.

In the first shot opposite, Catherine McNeil is not wearing false lashes. I have only applied a light layer of mascara to her eyes, as well as foundation and lipstick. Her makeup doesn't change over the following pages, only her lashes do. And you can see the difference in each shot.

Eyelash glue

Most eyelashes are sold with a complementary lash glue. But I would recommend that you buy a tube of professional eyelash glue, that is sold separately, from any quality makeup store, because these complementary glues don't adhere very well. In the false lash glue family, there are three types:

- **Standard glue**, which is white in colour and dries clear.
- **Waterproof and higher strength**, also white in colour and dries clear. I would recommend this glue for the heavy lash that needs more support.
- **Black eyelash glue**. I definitely recommend this when using a black liquid eyeliner or a black smoky eye shadow as it will be undetectable, unlike the clear-drying glue which you might be able to see with black.

natural lashes

On Catherine's first shot, I have applied a feathery single-strip lash. I call this the J.Lo lash, as she's known for it. With this lash, you can apply mascara either before or after you place it on your eyes. Just remember, the glue must be dry if you're applying mascara afterwards, because the slightest tension can pull the lash off.

These lashes are great for

- all eye shapes
- lifting the eyes
- opening the eye more; a tip here—apply mascara to the bottom lash as well (in this shot, I have applied mascara on top of the false lash and a subtle amount to the bottom lashes).

General tip

Whenever I'm doing shows and all the models are having the same makeup look using false lashes, even though the makeup is to look the same I find myself using completely different lashes to achieve this because of the different eye shapes. So my point is, remember that lashes are like shoes—you need to fit them; some will be too long, short, wide or heavy. A great way to check you have used the right ones is to look straight up, hold a mirror underneath and check that the false lash blends with yours, and that there are no gaps.

knot free flare long black

Lashes used here

flare under black

knot free medium black

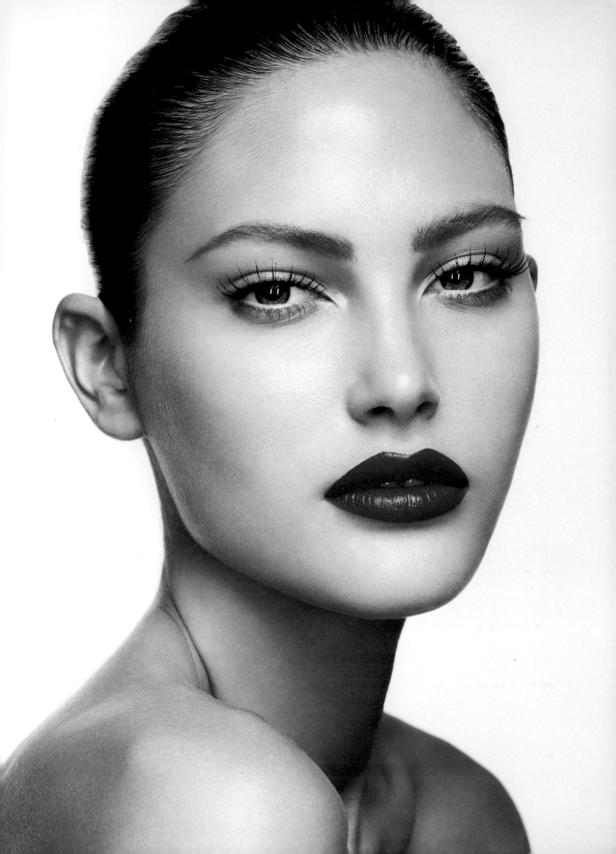

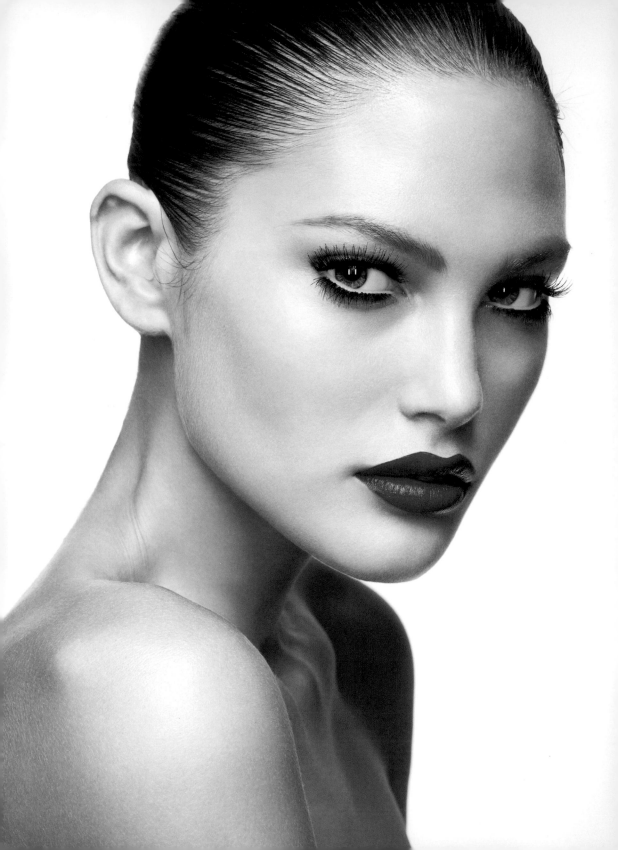

lux lashes

I call this look the 'eye-opener'. The best way to enlarge your eyes is to apply lashes to both top and bottom. Yes, I admit it's not easy to do, so let me take you through it step by step and give you great tips.

I like to apply all the single bottom lashes first (and after applying mascara). Why? Because when we blink, the lashes have a habit of sticking themselves to the top lash (very annoying and time-consuming).

There are two ways of applying bottom lashes: you either apply the glue 'under' the false lash then stick the lashes 'on top' of your natural lash, or you apply the glue 'on top' of the false lash then apply it 'under' your natural lash. A little confusing, I know, but you need to give this one a few goes to get it right.

Wait until all the lash glue has completely dried before you apply the top lashes or they will stick together. You can tell when the glue has dried because it goes clear (use white glue not black on the bottom lash).

Once you have achieved the bottom lash (and haven't ripped your hair out), the top is easy. Add a little glue to each individual lash, then apply one by one (as I have used individual lashes).

flare under black

General tips

When using single top lashes, apply them mostly to the outer corners as this lifts the eyes and gives them a sexy look.

You can use full-strip lashes underneath—just make sure they are not too long or too wide. There are so many on the market, you just need to find the best fit.

Lashes used here

high-impact lashes

This one speaks for itself. I have applied a heavy-strip lash; note that I haven't changed her makeup at all. Isn't it amazing what a lash can do? Apply mascara before putting on the lash, and keep the mascara to the top lash only, because it can start to look a little draggy!

These lashes are great for
- anyone who's game to wear them
- larger sized eyes
- Asian eyes.

These are not recommended for
- very rounded eyes
- small eyes
- eyes with few natural lashes (remember the false lashes need support).

General tip
Because this lash is extremely heavy, it needs support, so don't use one this thick if you have very few of your own lashes (see options on the left), because it will just keep dropping. And in most cases, you have to hold the lash up to your lash line and make sure the strip is not too long. Often, I will cut a few millimetres off the longest end of the false lash so it fits well, and apply extra glue especially on the ends.

Lashes used here

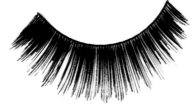 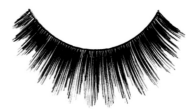

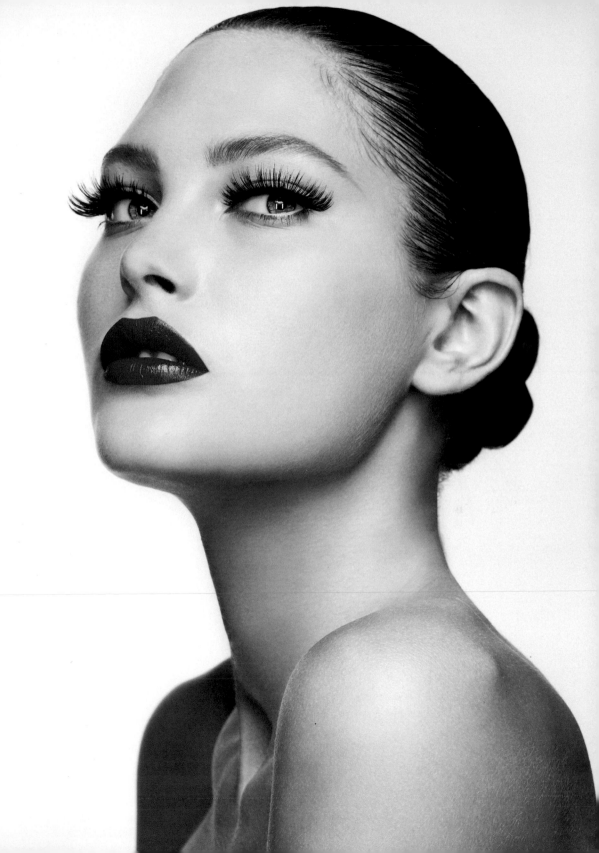

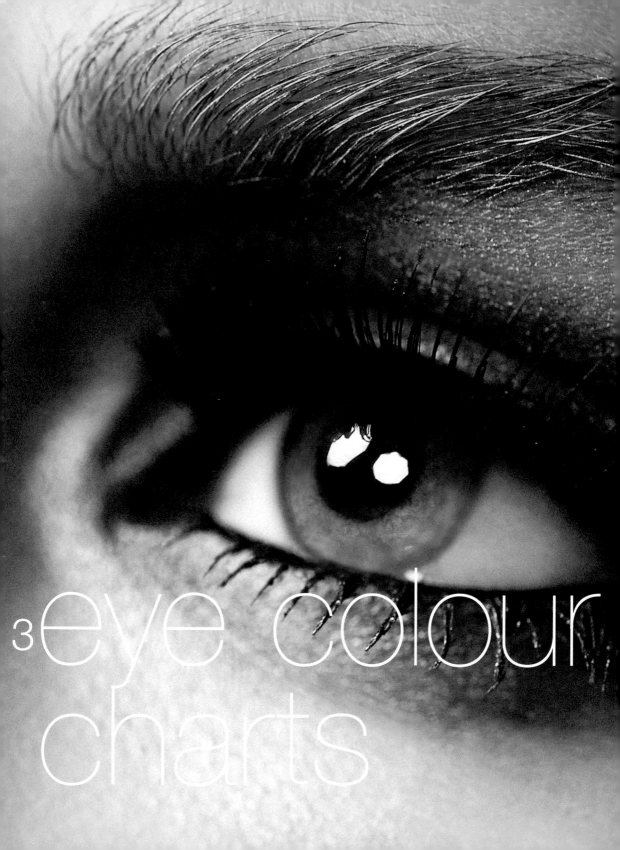

³eye colour charts

d o you know the number one question I get asked? 'What colour suits me?' (Actually, the number one question I get asked is 'Will you do the makeup for my wedding?' but 'What colour suits me?' is certainly a close second.) And although it's a great question (the colour one, not the wedding one), it's also a question which is very difficult to answer.

Why? Because half the time, the women asking me have got the wrong hair colour, the wrong-coloured clothing and the wrong accessories. And they are hoping that the 'right' lipstick will somehow magically pull the whole ensemble together.

Now, I am a makeup artist not a magician, and there is only so much that makeup can achieve. But what I will say is this: I believe wearing the wrong colour around your eyes is worse than wearing the wrong-coloured shirt (although I did see some shirts in Hawaii that nearly caused me to revise my opinion). And I dare say that if you get your makeup colours right, you can get away with wearing a coloured top that may not technically be one of your best or most flattering shades.

So because I take this topic very seriously, I consulted an expert in colour science. Bronwyn Fraser knows more about colour and the science of colour than anyone else I know, with years of experience working within the hair, beauty and fashion industries and also as a personal stylist. So you can trust that the following text is scientifically sound. (You can check out Bronwyn's website www.styleestablishment.com.au)

'There are no rules when it comes to fashion' … how often do we hear that quote? This is certainly true to an extent, as any makeup artist or fashion stylist will tell you, and the 'rules' are often broken to create a wow-factor or dramatic visual effect for magazine shoots or fashion shows. When it comes to selecting clothes, makeup, accessories or basically anything worn above the waist, the very first checkpoint for me is always colour, before cut, fit, style, fabric or anything else! Get the colour right and you are more than halfway there.

There are individual colours or colour families we can all wear to enhance and harmonise our natural colouring and emphasise our number one feature—our EYES! Always remember, your eyes are the first feature anyone sees when they look at your face, followed by your lips. To understand some easy colour basics when choosing your eye colours, refer to the eye colour charts in the following pages.

Highlighters/enhancers

These shades will really open up your eyes. You won't always find this written on the package but basically they are colours that highlight or reflect your own natural eye colour—don't worry we have worked that out for you in the colour charts.

Intensifiers/poppers

These colours, on an artist's colour wheel, are made of predominantly the opposite pigments to your own eyes, and therefore provide maximum contrast value to really brighten and illuminate your natural eye colour.

Neutrals

These are shades which are considered 'neutral' as they are made of varying combinations of the three primary colours, blue, red and yellow. There are warmer browns containing more yellow pigments that are suited to warmer brown, green and hazel eyes, and cooler browns containing more blue pigments best suited to deep brown, blue, cool green and cool hazel eyes, yet all do contain a combination of the three primary colours in their mix. Shades of brown eye shadow are universal and can be worn by anyone, any time, for a natural or sophisticated look depending on how it is applied.

Metallics

These high-shine reflective shades can be warm, cool or neutral and a little goes a long way! Metallic shades will draw maximum attention to wherever they are applied (many highlighters are metallic), so if your skin is less than perfect, be aware as metallics will highlight any flaws or fine lines. Used all over, they will give a beautiful, fresh sheen for both daytime and evening.

Accents

These are deep, vivid or bright colours used on either the upper or lower eye areas and are best applied in minimal quantities, such as a fine line very close to the lash line or a corner accent on either the inner and/or outer corners, for that extra impact. Think of these as 'accessory' shades, just like a great pair of shoes, handbag or earrings to complete a look.

blue eyes

Select your eye tone

Eye shadows

WARM BLUES	COOL BLUES	ALL BLUES
Best shadow for all warm blue-coloured eyes	Best shadow for all cool blue-coloured eyes	Shades to intensify and make all blue eyes 'pop'

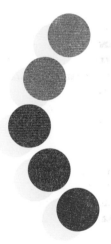

Eye-shadow pigments to highlight and enhance

ALL BLUE EYES

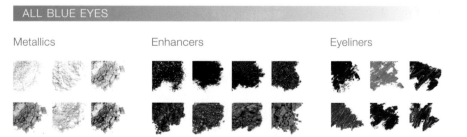

Metallics   Enhancers   Eyeliners

green eyes

Select your eye tone

ALL GREEN EYES

Eye shadows

WARM GREENS	COOL GREENS	ALL GREENS
Best shadow for all warm green-coloured eyes	Best shadow for all cool green-coloured eyes	Shades to intensify and make all green eyes 'pop'

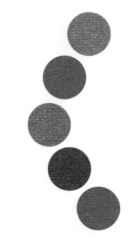

Eye-shadow pigments to highlight and enhance

ALL GREEN EYES

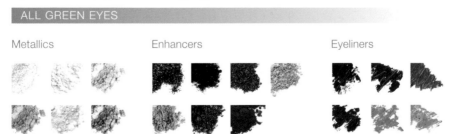

Metallics

Enhancers

Eyeliners

24

brown eyes

Select your eye tone

Eye shadows

WARM BROWNS
Best shadow for all warm
brown-coloured eyes

COOL BROWNS
Best shadow for all cool
brown-coloured eyes

ALL BROWNS
Shades to intensify and make
all brown eyes 'pop'

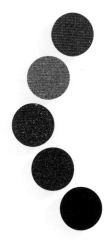

Eye-shadow pigments to highlight and enhance

ALL BROWN EYES

Metallics

Enhancers

Eyeliners

hazel eyes

Select your eye tone

Eye shadows

TRUE HAZELS	GOLDS	ALL HAZELS
Best shadow for all green/hazel-coloured eyes	Best shadow for all warm/golden hazel-coloured eyes	Shades to intensify and make all hazel eyes 'pop'

Eye-shadow pigments to highlight and enhance

ALL HAZEL EYES

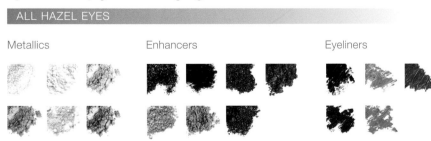

Metallics   Enhancers   Eyeliners

neutrals

These are considered neutral shades and can be worn by all eye colours, any time.

Eye shadows for all eye colours

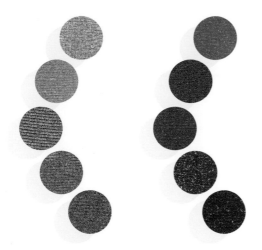

Eye-shadow pigments to highlight and enhance

ALL EYES

Metallics

Enhancers

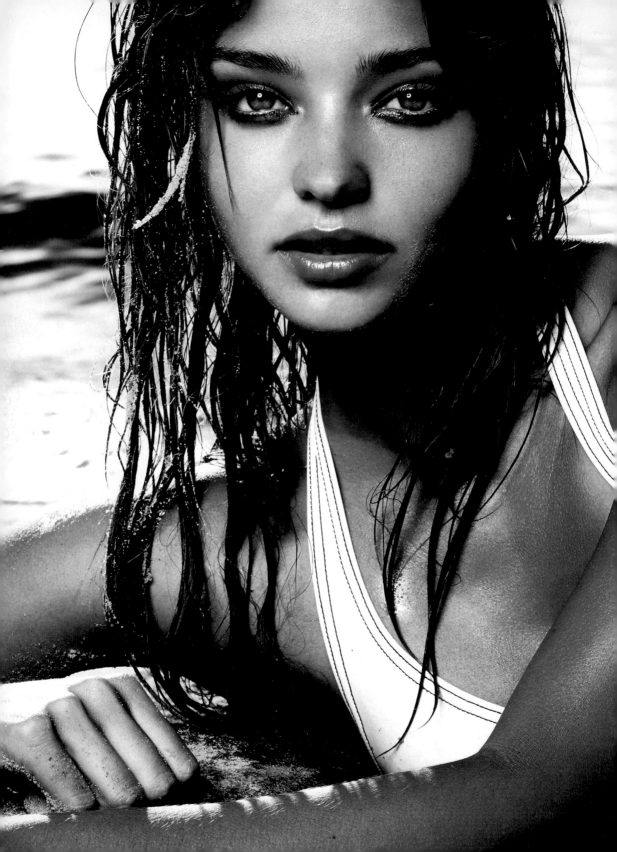

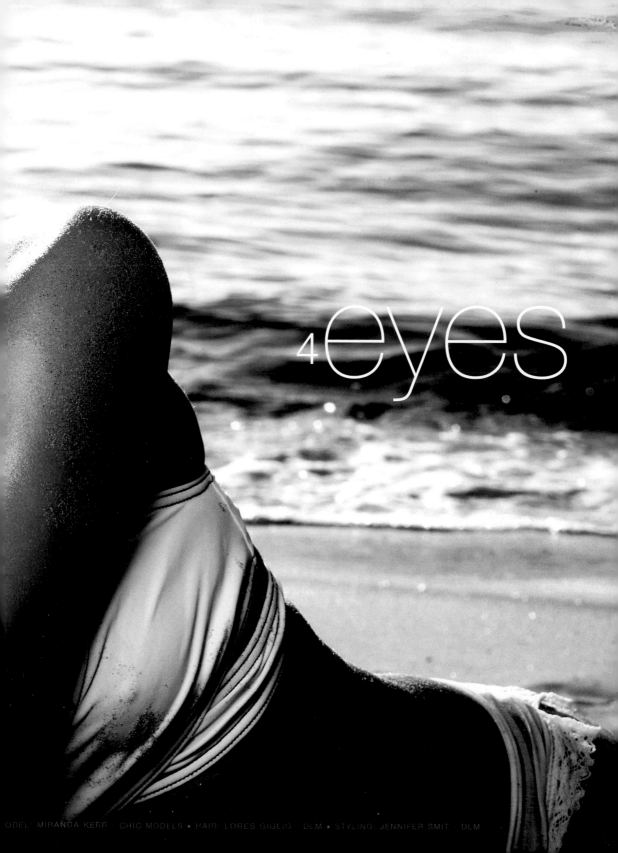

4eyes

MODEL: MIRANDA KERR - CHIC MODELS • HAIR: LORES GIGLIO - DLM • STYLING: JENNIFER SMIT - DLM

m

ost makeup books will tell you how to do the foundation first, and then how to conceal before you begin your eye makeup. But my philosophy is different. The eyes are the most powerful feature in the face, and I believe they should be done first.

Whether you have large, small, round, almond-shaped or Asian eyes, they are the first thing anyone notices. So how you tackle them, in a makeup sense, is crucial. The eyes are the key to successful makeup. They mirror all your efforts in trying to achieve a certain look. But more than that, they affect everything, including the overall shape of your face. If you get the eyes right, you've pretty much nailed it.

I do the eyes first for two main reasons. First, it avoids that nasty little thing known as 'fallout'. Fallout is that annoying eye shadow that continually drops on your cheeks, usually after you have applied your foundation, which you constantly have to wipe off. It wastes a lot of time and ruins your foundation. (Sorbolene cream is terrific for gently removing fallout.)

Second, I find that most women only allocate minimal time to do their makeup in the mornings, and yet they spend most of this time doing foundation! It doesn't make sense to put all your energy and effort into doing what's easy—the foundation—when you should be concentrating on what takes the longest and is the most intricate—your eyes. You can always do your foundation in the car on the way to work (I certainly do), on the train (most women will just think you're applying sunscreen anyway), or in the bathroom at work just before you enter the office.

If you do your eyes first, and you don't like how they look when you're done, then you can simply wipe it off and start again WITHOUT having to redo your base. But before you do any eye makeup, YOU MUST PREP YOUR EYES. Remember, your eyelids are one of the oiliest parts of your face, so please don't apply more oil to them. I've given you step-by-step instructions on how to prep your eyes (see page 34) so please use them!

How to achieve great eye makeup

Eye makeup is about knowing what you have, and knowing how to enhance it. Take a close look at your eyes and determine:

- what colour are they?
- what shape are they?
- what don't you like about your eyes?

The eye colour charts I've given you in this book (see pages 21–27) will help you work out which colours best suit your eyes. There's an amazing variety of eye shadows, pencils, mascaras, false eyelashes, etc., all designed to make you look fantastic. Keep on referring to the colour charts, especially as you consider new looks and colours, either at the makeup counter or as you read the book, and don't be afraid to experiment. In the case of the eyes, practice makes perfect.

Throughout this chapter, I talk about creating a wash over the eyelids. A wash is a primary colour, representing the tone you're going to use. If you're going to create eye makeup with a blue intensity, for example, you would begin with a wash of blue. It's purely a base of colour. Everything else is for the shape. A wash:

- can be soft or intense
- refers to the application, and is not a pastel beginning
- can be either dry or wet
- can be applied either to the middle lid or over the whole eyelid area
  (this is explained in every step-by-step in the following pages).

You'll also notice that I use metallic colours in this chapter. When using metallic colours on the lower lash line of the eyes, it's crucial to keep them very close to the lash line. If you let metallic colours drop too low, it will look like you haven't slept in weeks, it will magnify any fine lines and make them look worse, and will make you look like an old member of the Spice Girls. To top things off, it can also have a scaling effect. ALL TO BE AVOIDED.

Eye shape

The most common problem with eye shape is that often women don't know what to do to minimise or enhance a certain shape. Whatever your eye shape, my golden rule is to NEVER DO THINGS IN HALF on the eye. You should always extend lines and shadows either one-third or two-thirds of the way. If you do anything halfway across, it cuts the eye in half and makes it look distorted.

So let's address the biggest problems with shape:

If you have small eyes

You can make them look larger. The best trick in the book is to curl your lashes (apply mascara, of course), and apply creamy white pencil (not waterproof) to the inner rim. This creates an illusion of larger eyes. If you feel confident, adding single false lashes to the top outer lash line will also enlarge the eyes (see the False Eyelashes chapter, page 9).

If you have very large, rounded or protruding eyes

Never use hard-edged eyeliner, either above or below; a smudged liner is the only type allowed. Hard-edged liner results in framing the eye and bringing attention to the roundness. I love to make this eye shape more cat-like by applying dark pencil to the inner rim of the eye; this helps to shrink the eye shape. Keep all dark colours to the outer third corner of the eye, and if you want to create a smoky effect don't follow the natural shape of the eye; the outline should be more of a square shape—the trick is to make the eye shadow into a more rectangular shape—i.e. don't follow the natural roundness of the eye—and to extend the outer corner of the eye. Don't highlight the middle of the eyelid, and only apply mascara to the top lashes.

If you have heavy eyelids

Whatever colour you choose as your eye shadow, use it in the inner corners (top and bottom) of your eyes. This way, if your eyes are open, you can still see the colour on your lids (i.e. it won't get covered by the heavy lid). Eyebrow shape is essential; anything too arched will accentuate heavy lids, so you want a straighter brow shape with a slight arch. No frosty eye shadow allowed for heavy eyelids (see *Kath & Kim* for reference)! However, using a matt contouring shade on the lids is a great way of giving the illusion of a deeper set socket.

If you have close-set eyes

The best tip is to use highlighter in the inner corners. Any darkening or shading or smoking is to be restricted to the outer corner of the eye—this includes keeping the false eyelashes on the outer corner. So the basic rule is that everything that is light or highlighting or metallic goes on the inner part of the eye and anything dark or smoky goes on the outer part of the eye, to 'wing' it out. If you darken the eye the whole way across, you actually make the problem more obvious.

If you have very small eyelashes

The solution is easy—use false lashes! I've given you a whole chapter on this, and I've used them in almost every step-by-step in this chapter, so there's no excuse!

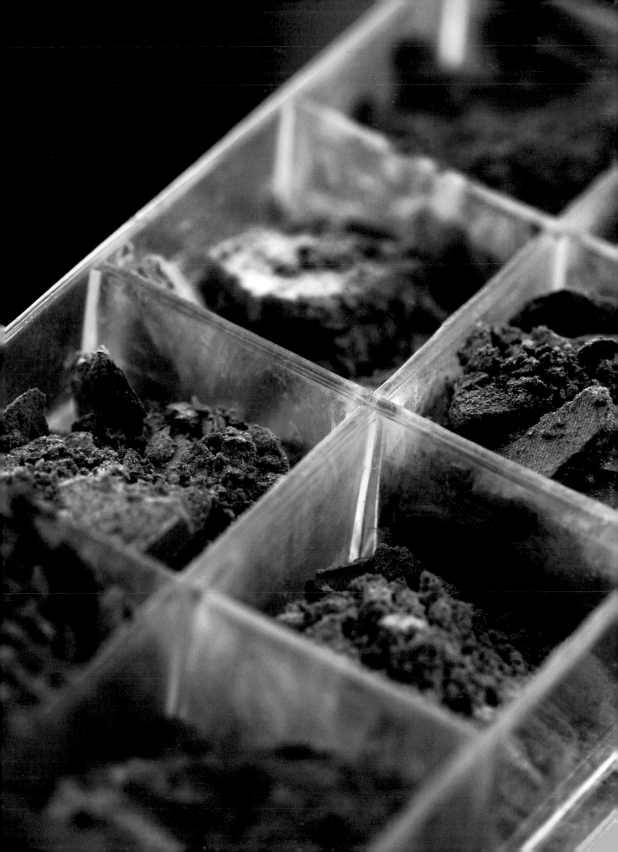

step-by-step eye prep

Most women don't realise that the eyelids are one of the oiliest parts of the face. If you don't believe me, go ahead and wipe your eyelids. You will find the same kind of oil you would find in your T-zone.

Oil is the number one killer of eye shadow. So all oil must be removed from your eyelids before applying eye shadow. The only time I don't remove oil is when I want greasy eyes for a photo shoot.

If you have some doubts about this, try this little experiment. Prep one eye according to the steps below, and then apply eye shadow. Then apply eye shadow to your other eye as you would normally do, without prepping, and watch the difference in the way your eye makeup lasts on your prepped eye. I never retouch eye makeup, even on a twelve-hour shoot, because I always prep the eyes properly.

Step 1
Cleanse your lids with a water-based cleanser. You can also use alcohol- and perfume-free baby wipes—that's what I use on every shoot. Do not moisturise your eyelids afterwards.

Step 2
The biggest question: do I apply foundation to the eyelids or don't I? My answer is yes, absolutely, every single time. Why? Because your eyelids, if you look closely at them, have blue and red tones or tinges. When you apply foundation, you knock out all the blue–red tones, giving you a great neutral canvas to allow your eye shadows to be true to their colour. (To test the true colour of your eye shadow, particularly if it's your favourite, apply a swatch of it to the back of your hand, and another swatch to your fingertip. And look at the difference in colour.) And remember, all foundations contain a moisturiser of some kind. This is all the moisture you will need on your eyelids.

Step 3
Lightly powder the eyelids with translucent powder. You can do this with a cotton pad. Powder will go cakey (not what you want) if you have too much oil or moisturiser on your lids.

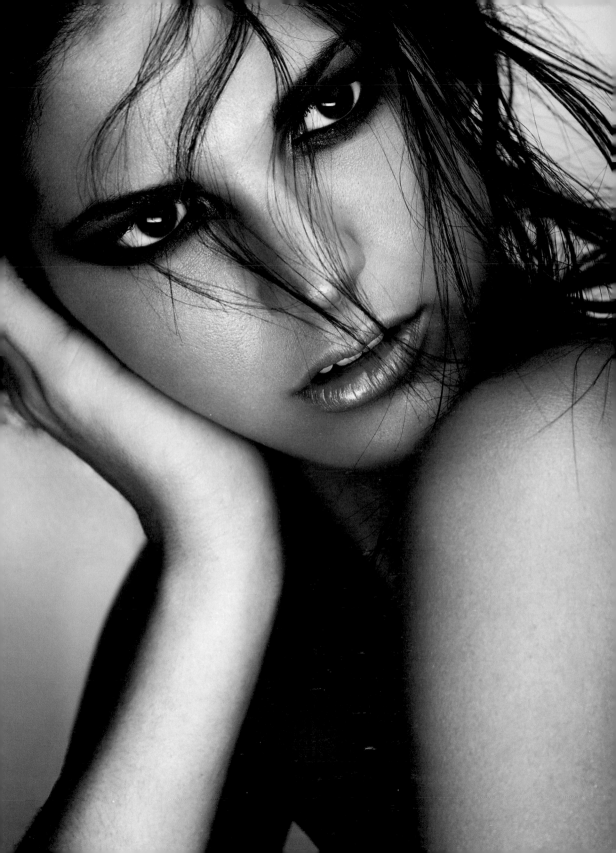

smoky eyes

1 Prep the eye and powder lightly; this will help with the blending. Apply a smoky chocolate-brown shadow under the eye. Keep the shape slightly rounded (as shown).

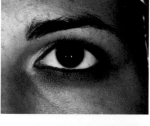

2 Using a large brush, apply a soft wash of the same colour to the whole lid, all the way up to the brow bone, and extend out to the edge of the eye.

TIP

When you're applying the black pencil to the eye, pull it out and don't let it stop suddenly. Don't let it look too square.

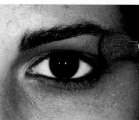

3 Apply a heavy black kohl pencil to the inside rim of the eye and also messily above the whole top lash line, pulling the line out slightly. Heat up the pencil by rubbing it on the back of your hand, and blend the line above the top lashes.

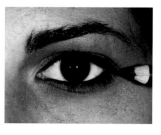

4 Mix black with khaki eye shadow and smudge it around the whole eye, close to the lash line. Use a small rounded brush to blend.

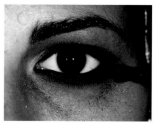

5 Wet the brush, and smudge the black/khaki shadow up towards the brow bone. Don't worry if the line isn't perfect, as you will be blending another colour with it all the way up to the brow bone.

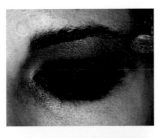

6 Apply an aubergine eye shadow all the way under the brow, blending it to soften the black edges.

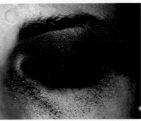

7 Clean up under the eye. Apply your foundation base. Use corn-silk powder to blend the black under the eye. Curl lashes, then apply a full set of false lashes. It is very important to define the brows with this look. Finish with a metallic green shadow in the inner corner of the eye.

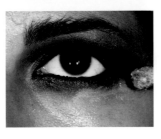

LASHES USED

TIPS

Lining the inner eye with a creamy white pencil will open up the eyes.

Lining the eyes with black gives you a cat-like effect.

You can't go past deep violet tones for smoky eyes, especially when you're wearing black.

There is no eye shape that is not suited to smoky eyes.

If you want to add a little more colour, just hit the inner corner of your eyelids with a bright lavender, gold or blue. Metallic colours are best.

Smoky eyes are fantastic for women with small lips; focusing on the eyes takes the attention off the lips.

If done properly, smoky eyes don't have to be touched up after the initial application.

Remember, they don't have to be black and dark. You can achieve smoky eyes with bronzed colours, a jewelled effect, and even shades of green.

bronzed eyes

TIPS

Because you're applying the eye shadow wet, you must not look up for at least 30 seconds, as it will cause the makeup to crease.

Using an antique gold as opposed to a yellow gold looks more elegant.

Use powder on the eyelid to blend the rest of the eye shadow.

Once your eye is complete, take the same gold you used on the lid and apply to the inner corner of the eye and to the cupid's bow of your lips.

For a more dramatic look, apply single/individual false lashes to the outer corners of the upper lash line.

The gold and bronze colour palettes look amazing on blue eyes.

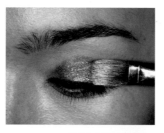

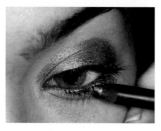

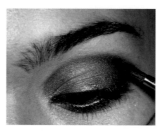

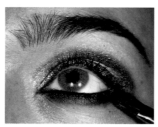

1 Prep the eyelid, making sure it is well powdered all around; this will help you to blend eye shadows better. Using a wet medium brush, apply antique gold eye shadow to the entire eyelid. Wetting the brush will minimise fallout and intensify the gold.

2 Overload the inner rim of the eye with an antique gold eye pencil—don't be afraid to load it up. Make sure the pencil you use is not waterproof. Eye pencil used in the inner rim disappears quickly due to blinking, etc., so ensure constant reapplication for a lasting look.

3 Using a smaller brush, finely apply a rusty brown eye shadow along the socket line. If you find this isn't blending, then go back to the first step and powder well. Intensify the brown shadow in the outer corner of the eye.

4 Apply the same rusty brown eye colour all the way along the lower lash line. Curl lashes using a curler, and apply lots of jet-black mascara to both top and bottom lashes.

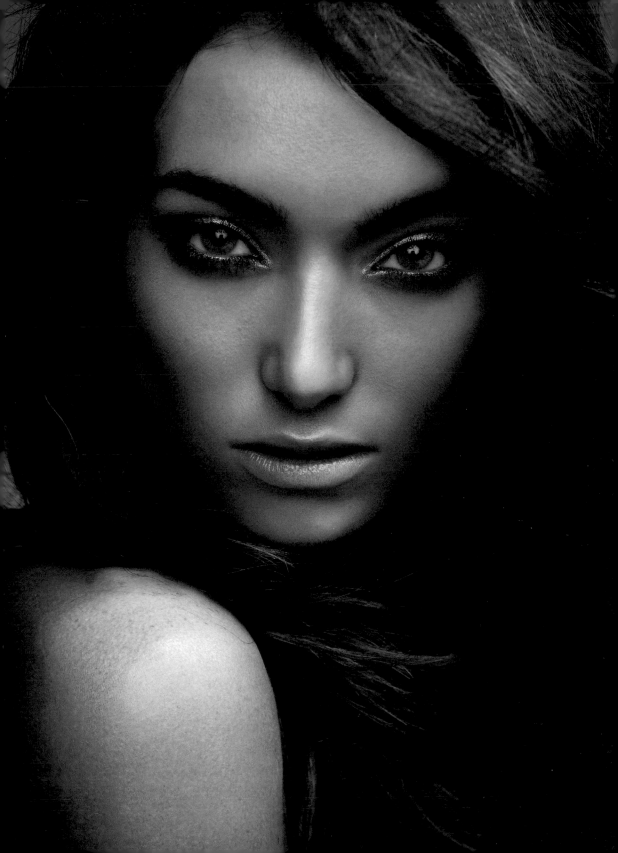

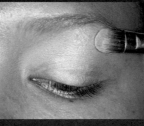

1 Using a pure white pencil, apply heavily to the inner eye rim. (Note: you will have to apply this again at the end.) Using a pearlised (has a pearl reflection) gold eye shadow, apply to the middle of the eyelid, then carry it right up to the brow bone.

TIPS

This eye shadow is not recommended for puffy eyelids, however, if you are using for puffy lids don't carry it all the way up to the brow bone. Instead, stop just above the lid.

If you have blonde lashes, wear brown mascara.

If you don't want such a heavy-lashed effect, apply a thick coating of brown mascara without using the false eyelashes.

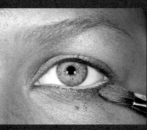

2 Apply a lavender eye shadow from the inner corner of the eye socket, blending up to the eyebrow and along the lower lash line. Make sure you keep the lid golden and don't carry the lavender too far across the upper lid.

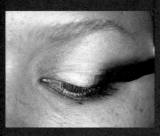

3 Smudge a little black kohl pencil into the top outer corner of the eye. Load up a small brush with dark violet eye shadow and blend it up and out as shown. Notice the eye is never closed—this gives you a smoother finish and stops the eye shadow from creasing.

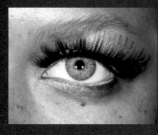

4 Because gold and lavender are such soft colours, I have strengthened the look by using full, strong, brown (not black) false eyelashes. Notice the little bit of white along the lash line. It's eyelash glue that will dry in 5 minutes (it's white when it's wet, clear when dry).

MODEL: LARA BINGLE • HAIR: KAREN HOPWOOD - DLM

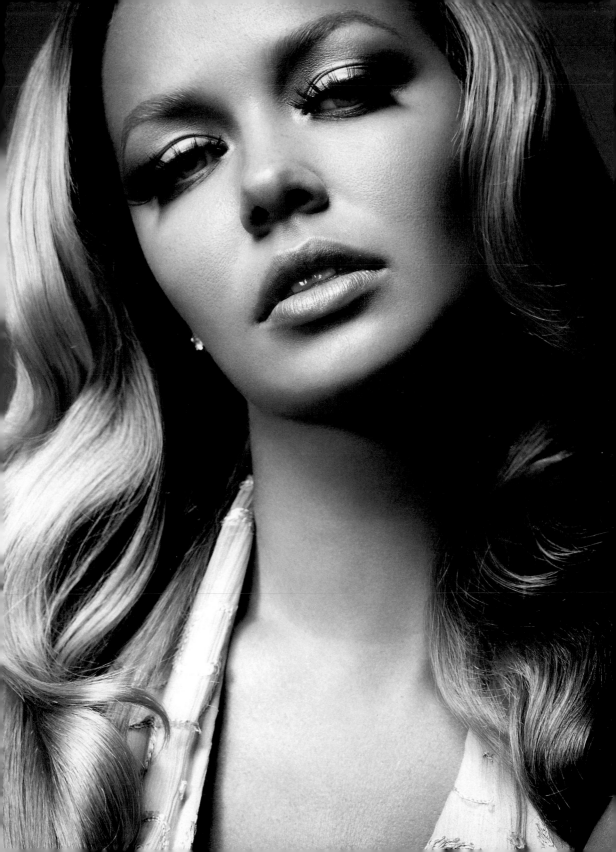

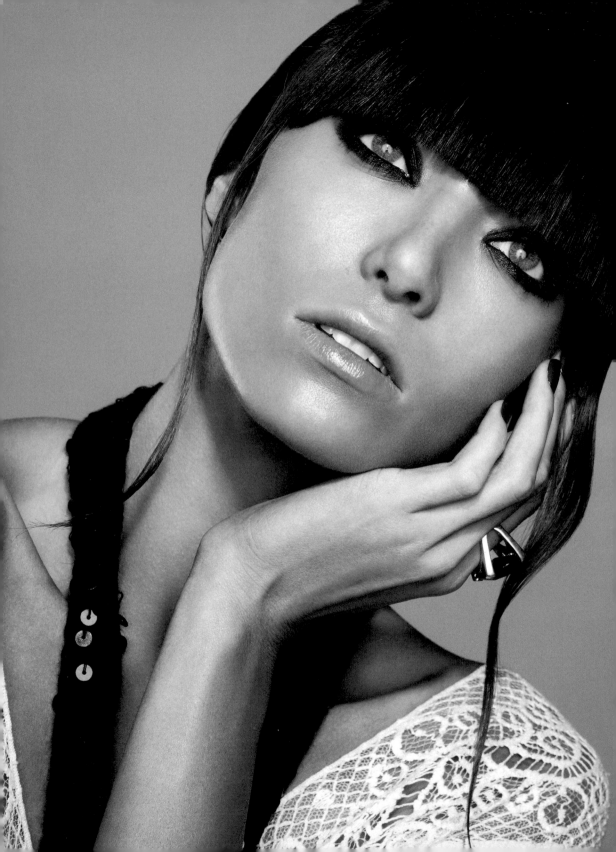

rock chick eyes

1 Apply an intense black kohl pencil or cream eyeliner to the inner rim and cover the entire eyelid; smudge with your finger. When lining the lower outer corner of the eye, smudge the pencil into and just below the lash line. The colour must be jet-black, otherwise it'll look dirty.

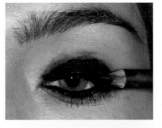

2 Using translucent powder that matches your skin tone, apply to the rest of the eye socket up to the brow bone. This will make the next stage much easier to blend.

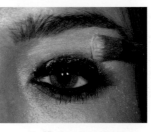

TIPS

Black fallout is hard to remove, even with the best of makeup removers. As well as Sorbolene, you can also use a water-based moisturiser under the eye to prevent staining.

Clumpy black mascara is hot with this look.

A high-shine luminescent foundation complements this look.

Use a translucent powder under the eye, below the black.

3 Dab some Sorbolene cream under the eye to make removing any dropped shadow easier (and avoid rubbing the skin). Using a small brush, apply dark metallic midnight-blue pigment to blend the black and lift the shape higher to just under the brow bone.

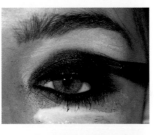

4 Apply the blue metallic pigment to the inner corner of the eye and underneath the lower lash line. Finish by applying lots of black mascara to the top and bottom lashes.

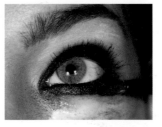

techno eyes

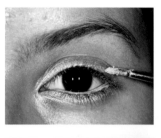

1 Prep the eyes and powder well. Using a fine brush, apply a soft metallic pale-gold shimmer powder over the entire eye, keeping it close to the lash line. Then apply a non-waterproof white pencil to the inner rim of the eye.

TIP

Gold leaf can be tricky as it sticks like glue. Only use a brush to pick it up from the packaging, otherwise it will stick to your fingers.

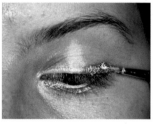

2 Using a medium brush, apply the same colour in the centre of the eyeball (as shown). This adds a beautiful highlight that will be visible when you blink.

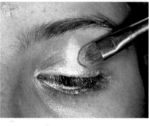

3 Using a wet fine brush, then apply a gold leaf (available from selected makeup stores and art shops) to the inner corner of the eye, and over the outer corner of the upper lid.

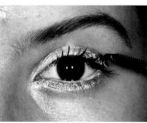

4 Curl lashes and apply a heavy amount of mascara to the top lashes only. Do not comb out your lashes, keep them clumpy.

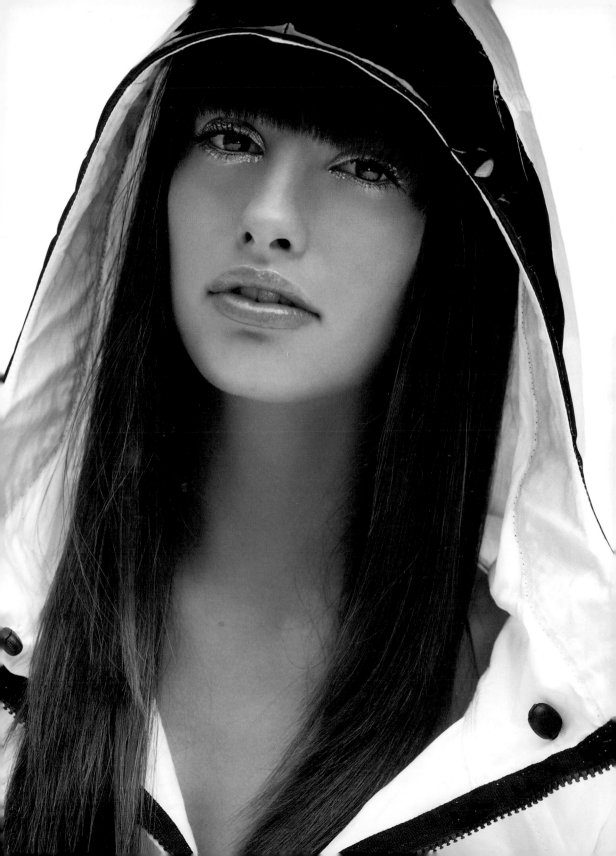

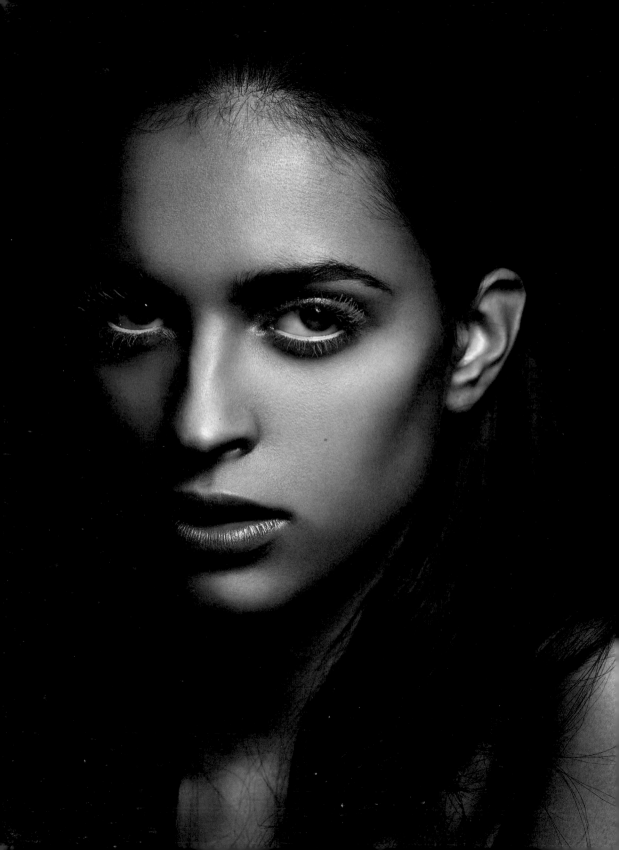

turquoise evening eyes

1 Using a medium brush, apply a soft mint-green wash to the whole eyelid, to just underneath the brow bone. Remember, this will blend easily if your eyelids are prepped and powdered.

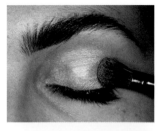

2 Using a thin brush, apply the same colour under the length of the bottom lash line. The colour must stay very close to the lash line, because if you let metallic colours drop too low it will look like you haven't slept in weeks, make fine lines look worse and have a scaling effect.

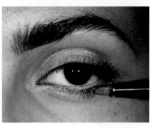

TIP

With this look, tone down blush so that it's virtually undetectable. This is a great look for low-light locations, awesome on dark-coloured eyes and all blue-toned eyes.

3 Apply a white pencil heavily to the inner rim of the eye. This makes your eyes look whiter, wider and more alive. Using a thin brush, apply a strong electric-blue pigment along the top and bottom outer lash line. Don't worry about fallout—fix it later.

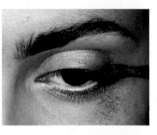

4 Curl lashes, and apply an intense amount of turquoise mascara. Using a fine angled brush, highlight the inner corners with soft iridescent silver.

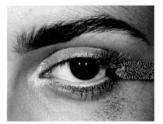

electric blue eyes

TIPS

The smaller the area you're working on, the smaller the brush should be.

Pale blue eye shadow can be very scary. If used incorrectly, it can look cheap and nasty. I believe most frosty eye shadow needs depth and intensity to look beautiful, so use a little black or a darker version of the colour you choose. With Michelle's eyebrows, I filled them in lightly to give more definition.

For step 3, you can also use black eye shadow along the lash line to make the colour more intense.

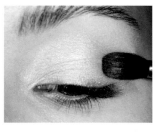

1 Prep the eyes and apply a soft wash of translucent powder. Using a medium brush, apply a soft, iridescent blue eye shadow to the whole eyelid and blend up to the brow bone.

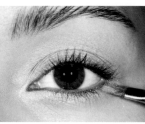

2 Using a small brush, apply the same colour all the way along the bottom of the eye. Make sure you use very light pressure; this will guarantee a smooth, even result. It helps to look up while doing this because it stretches the skin and stops unwanted lines from appearing.

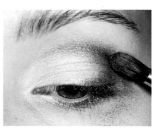

3 Using a medium brush, apply a midnight-blue shadow to create depth. Blend lightly under the brow bone and apply one-third of the way along the lash line. This should be the darkest point of the eye. Make sure to avoid gaps of bare skin and don't put too much pressure on the brush, as you will create fine lines.

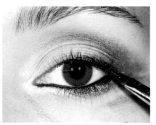

4 Apply a midnight-blue eye pencil, or cream eyeliner, heavily to the inner rim of the eye, and to the outer corner of the lid. This lifts the eye and makes it look younger and more cat-like. It also frames the eye, giving it more definition. Finish by applying mascara.

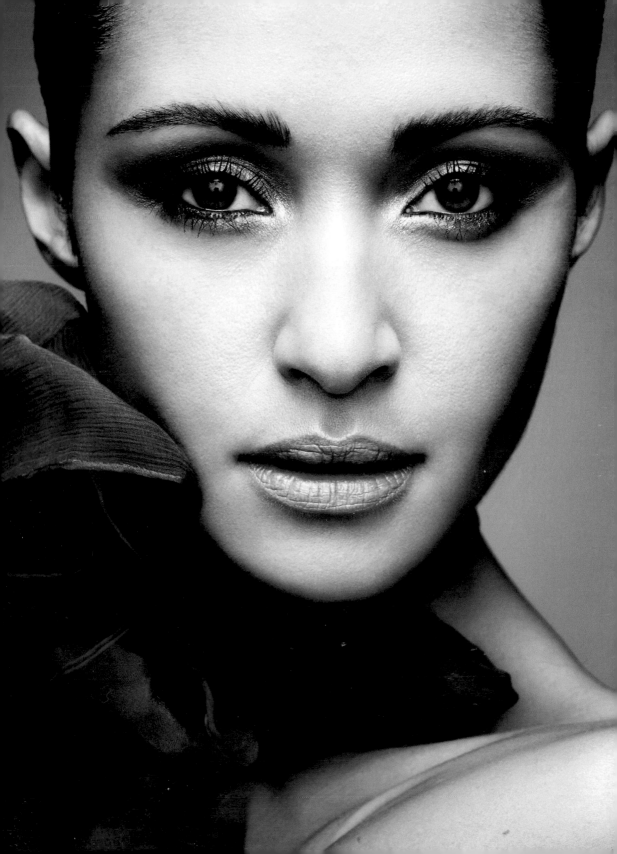

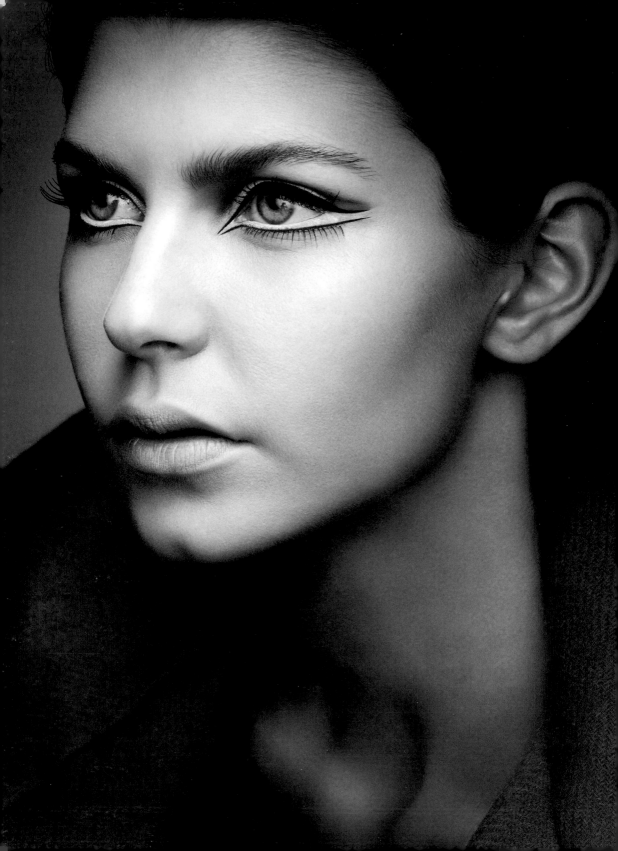

retro eyes

1 Lightly foundation the eyelid, but do not powder yet. Using a medium brush, apply white water-based liquid eye paint to the lid. Keep looking down while waiting for the paint to dry, otherwise it will crease. To set this, use a white eye shadow over the dried paint.

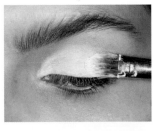

2 Heavily apply a white eye pencil to the inner rim of the eye. This needs to be non-waterproof to ensure an intense colour. Extend the white line straight out past the outer corner of the eye and create a triangle to the inner corner (as shown).

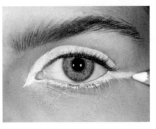

3 Using a stiff angled brush, apply black eye shadow above the eyelid (don't use a fine eyeliner brush). Extend the line out from the edge of the lid. Eyeliner looks its best when the line thickens towards the outer socket.

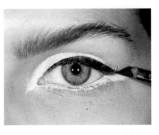

4 Using black eye shadow and a slightly wet angled brush, draw a line underneath the eye as shown, making sure you are looking directly ahead to ensure a straight line.

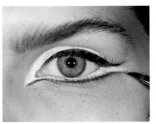

TIPS

The reason I am using a paint before the eye shadow is because eye shadows on their own don't give a strong enough intensity. You need to have the paint base to make the white stand out more. This is one of the most difficult looks to achieve. It will take at least half an hour to do.

Use a non-waterproof pencil on the inner rim of the eye because it is a wet area. A waterproof pencil will scratch the skin and will not work.

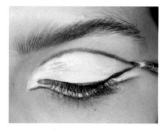

5 Extend the line above the top lash line up and out. Draw another thin line following the crease in the eyelid, moving from the inner to the outer, connecting to the line above the lid in the shape of a V.

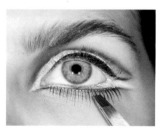

6 Using a thin brush, slightly blend the line into the crease in your lid.

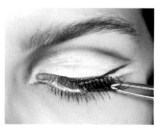

7 I am using clear eyelash glue on the bottom false lashes before applying mascara, which I rarely do. Apply a full set of lashes along the line you have created under the eye.

8 Apply a full set of false lashes to the top lash line, gluing it to the line you have already created with the eyeliner. Finish by applying mascara.

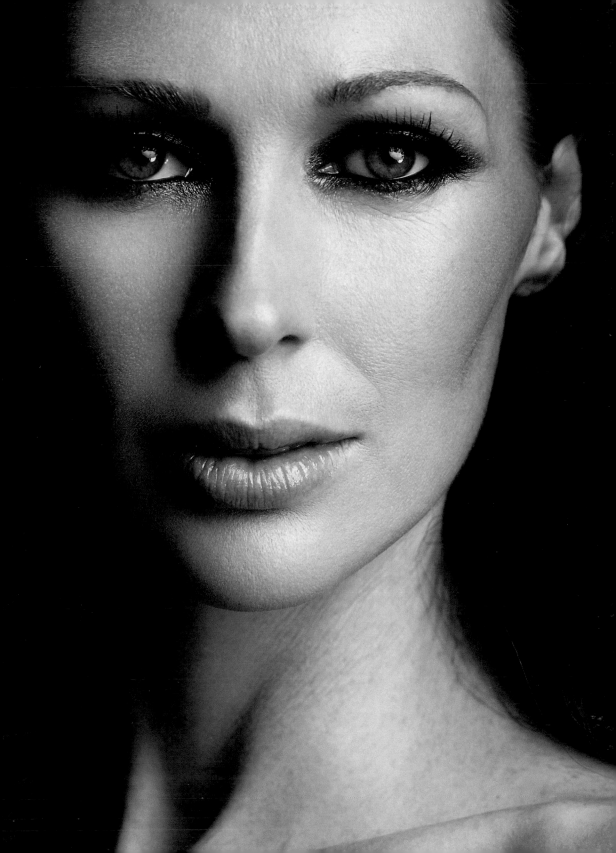

sexy eyes for redheads

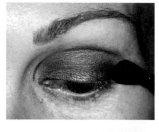

1 Prep the eyes. Using a medium brush, apply a purple wash over the whole eyelid, stopping just under the brow bone.

TIP

Make sure your brushes are very soft, and use a gentle motion. Harsh movements will create heavy lines, and make it harder to blend.

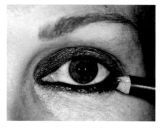

2 Using a wet angled brush, apply a copper pigment to the inner corners of the eye, top and bottom. Using the same brush (no need to clean it), apply an intense mahogany-red shadow under the bottom eyelashes, and in the inner corner of the eye, top and bottom.

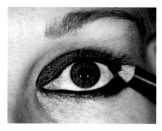

3 Line the eye rim heavily with a black non-waterproof eye pencil. This automatically changes the shape of the eye.

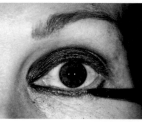

4 Line the upper rim of the eyelid heavily with the same non-waterproof black pencil.

5 Using a black shadow, heavily smudge the outer corner of the lid. Fill a clean medium brush with translucent powder, and use it to blend the black eye shadow and soften hard edges in an upward motion. This technique helps to extend the black into the outer corner of the eye.

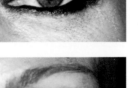

6 Clean up underneath the eye. The gentlest way to do this is to apply Sorbolene cream under the eye then use a wipe to remove any fallout.

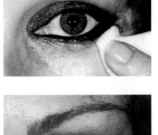

7 Curl lashes, and apply black mascara to the top and bottom lashes heavily (don't apply mascara if you are using false lashes—see the next step).

8 If you are using false lashes, apply a full set. Make sure they fit the eye correctly, and cut if necessary (for more information on applying lashes, refer to pages 9–19). Apply mascara. Notice the outer corner of the eye is not yet blended (blend after you apply your foundation).

TIPS

Heavy black pigments are hard to find. A lot of them end up looking grey. If you have trouble finding one, use a cream black eyeliner or pencil.

A great idea before you start your lips is to load them up with lanolin or lip balm so they are moist for when you are ready to apply lipstick.

If you use too many products (eye cream, sunscreen etc.) around the eyes, the eye shadow will get cakey and heavy.

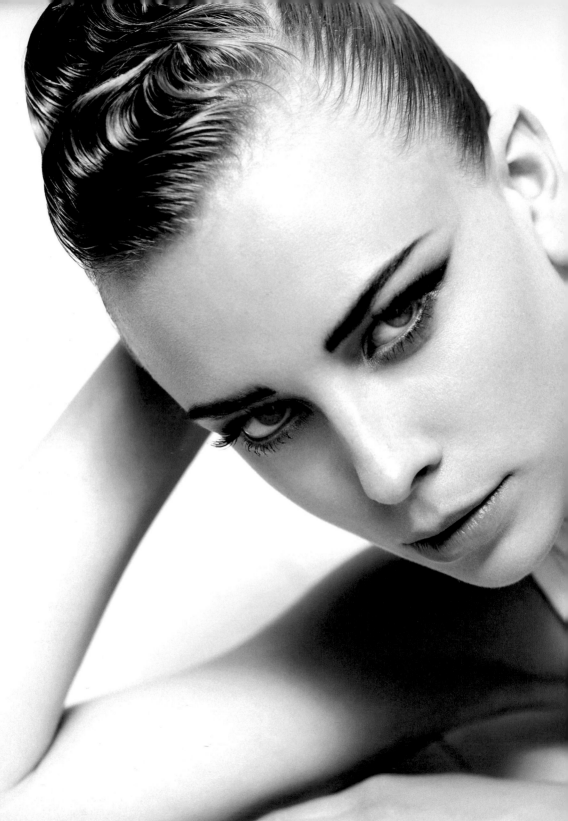

exotic eyes

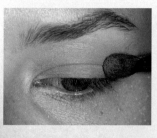

1 Prep the eyes. Using a medium brush, apply bright mustard-yellow eye shadow to the entire eyelid. Take the yellow softly up to the brow bone.

2 Using a medium round brush, apply a mahogany shadow along the entire socket line to the edge of the eye. Reapply the mustard yellow over this and use to blend with the mahogany.

3 Using a wet small brush, apply a black eye shadow to the outer corner of the eye and make a triangle shape by pulling out the black, then soften the edges (as shown).

TIP
Because this is such a strong and unique look, make sure you match it with prominent brows.

4 Apply strong turquoise eyeliner to the inner rim of the eye. Define brows. I have decided to keep the brow shape more straight here. Apply a full set of false lashes, and black mascara to both top and bottom lashes.

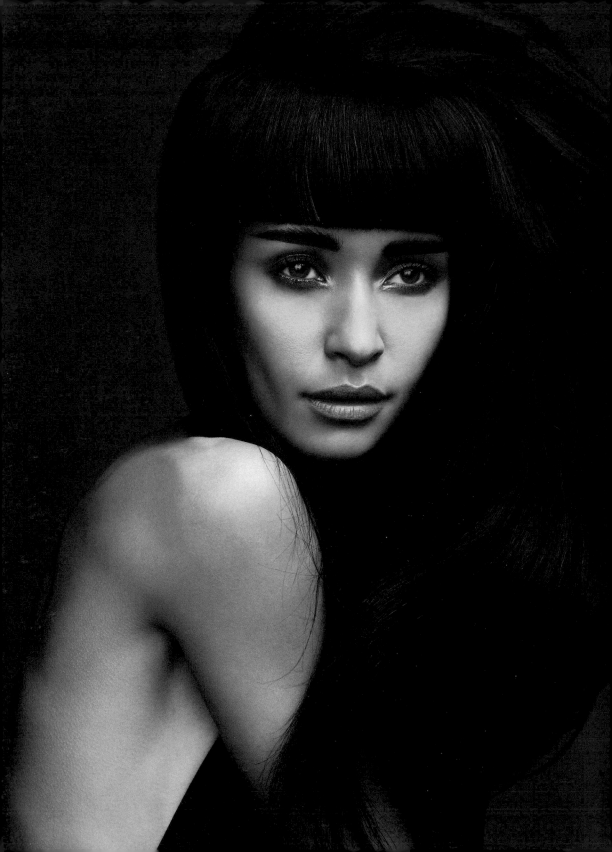

harajuku eyes

1 Create a stencil with sticky tape (use soft, magic tape which is easy to remove) directly under the eyebrow, to create a straight line (as shown).

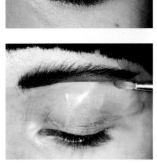

2 Use a deep-red eye shadow to draw in the area above the stencil line, to recreate the eyebrow. Then using a thin brush, apply a strong orange pigment along the brow line. Do not blend with the eye shadow. Then remove the tape.

3 Using a large brush (for easy blending), apply a cream khaki-coloured eye shadow all over lid. Do not extend it to the brow bone.

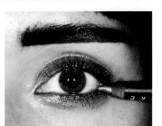

4 Apply gold eyeliner to the inner rim of the eye, and finish up with a coat of mascara. You can use mascara on the top and bottom lashes to keep a more rounded shape.

TIPS

To contrast with the shiny eyelids, I have used a sheer powder on the face—you don't want shiny skin with shiny eyes.

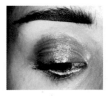

I've included this shot especially to show the problems created with grease and cream shadows. This shot was taken 10 minutes after makeup was applied; see how quickly the eye shadow has creased? Magazines are filled with wet, sexy-looking eyes, but these have a lasting ability of only 10 minutes. So only use if you are ready to constantly smooth it out.

egyptian eyes

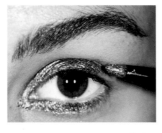

1 Using a wet small brush, apply a mahogany, deep chocolate-brown eye shadow underneath the eye and over the top lid, keeping the intensity in the inner corner.

TIP

Mahogany is the only colour in the colour wheel that is both cool and warm. It is suitable for any time of day and with any look. Gemma's brows are beautifully arched, however, to give a sexier, more polished look. Make the brows less rounded for a straighter look.

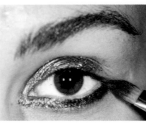

2 Using a small brush, apply the same shadow under the rim of the eye, then pull it out slightly to the outer edge of the eye to create a smudged eyeliner.

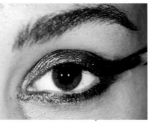

3 Turn your brush upside down, and apply the same shadow to the top lid. This will keep the intensity along the lash line (this will eliminate the mistake of leaving skin gaps). Apply more shadow to keep it heavier on the outer corner of the top lid.

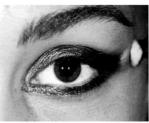

4 Apply a bit of loose translucent powder, making sure it matches your skin tone. In Gemma's case, I am using a yellow tone. Curl the lashes, and apply lots of mascara to top and bottom lashes. Clean up under the eye, and apply foundation.

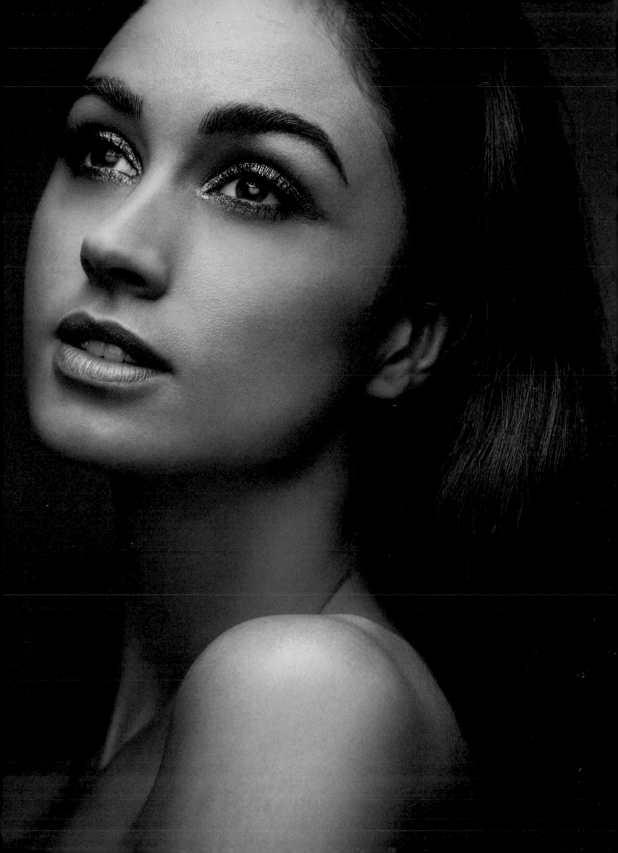

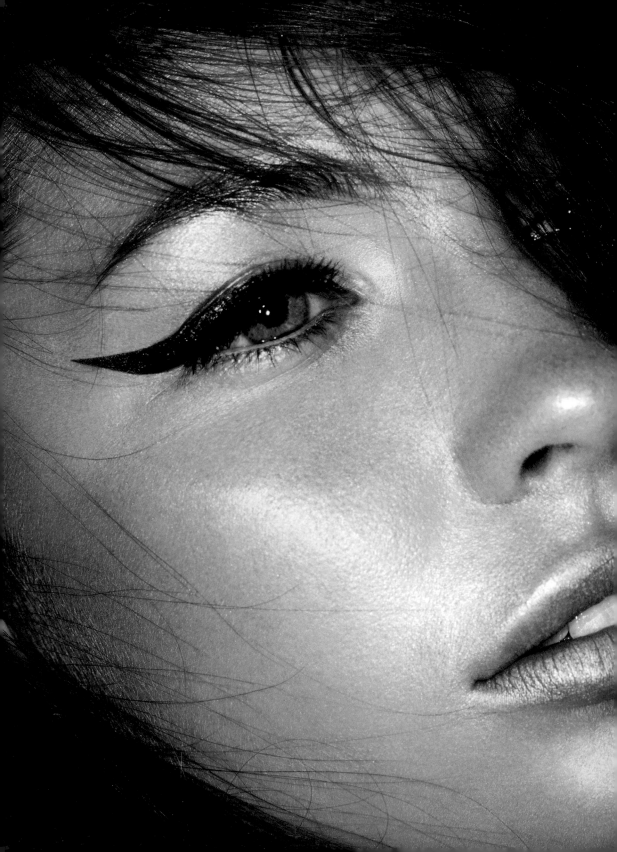

cat-like eyes

1 Imagine a line from the corner of your nose to the outer corner of your eye that continues to your temple. Your eyeliner needs to follow this angle. Apply sticky tape as a stencil on that angle. Using a small angled brush, apply black liquid liner along your lash line, flicking up onto the tape.

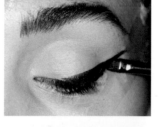

2 Wait for the liner to dry, then carefully peel off the tape. Apply a bright blue pigment on the inner corner of the eye, to meet the liquid liner.

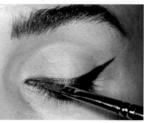

TIPS

The sticky tape will ensure your line is straight.

If you wish, you can use black eye shadow instead of the liquid liner.

3 Curl lashes and apply lots of mascara to the top lashes only; make sure the mascara is applied all the way to the bed of the lashes.

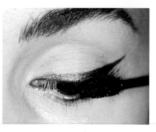

4 Apply false lashes to the top eyelid. Finish the look by applying foundation and a light metallic lipstick.

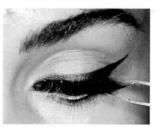

aqua eyes

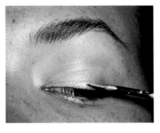

1 Prep your eyes and lightly powder. I am breaking the eyeliner into two sections. Using an eyeliner brush, apply an aqua-green eyeliner from the inside of the eyelid, stopping in the centre. This will stretch the skin and minimise wrinkles and creasing in the lid.

TIPS

This is one of the few dramatic eye looks where you can do the foundation first. Then use an alcohol-free baby wipe to remove oil from the eyelid. This will stop the eyeliner from bleeding.

Most liquid eyeliners tend to crack, so choose gel or cream liners instead. These will give you time to move and blend before they dry.

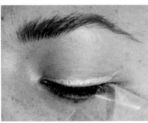

2 Apply sticky tape as a stencil on an imaginary angle, from the corner of your nose to the outer corner of your eye. Then finish applying the eyeliner from the centre to the upper outer edge as shown. The sticky tape will ensure you get a perfect line.

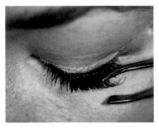

3 Curl lashes and apply lots of black mascara to the top and bottom lashes. Make sure the mascara is jet-black. Then apply a full lash that has been cut in half to the top lashes only (see the False Eyelashes chapter, page 9).

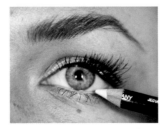

4 Apply non-waterproof white eyeliner to the inner rim of the eye. This will open up the eye and make it look more alive.

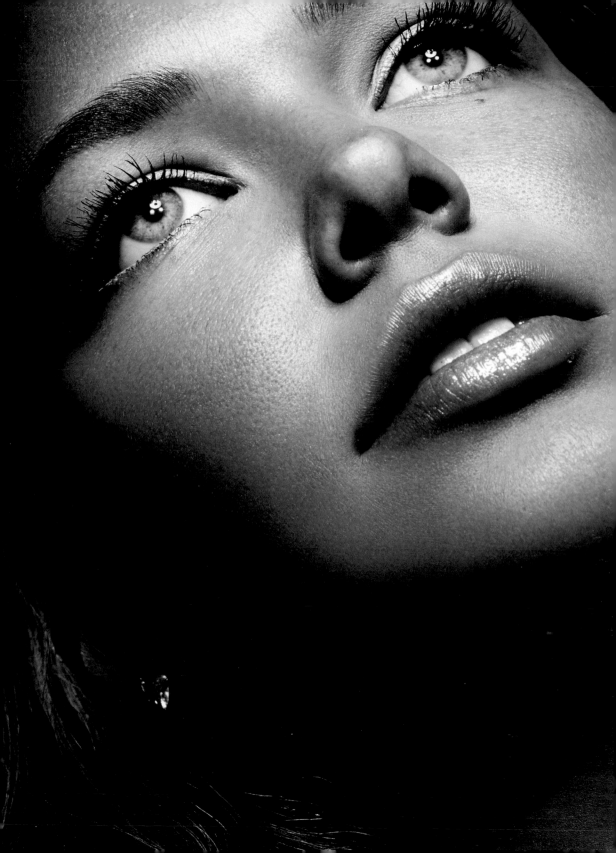

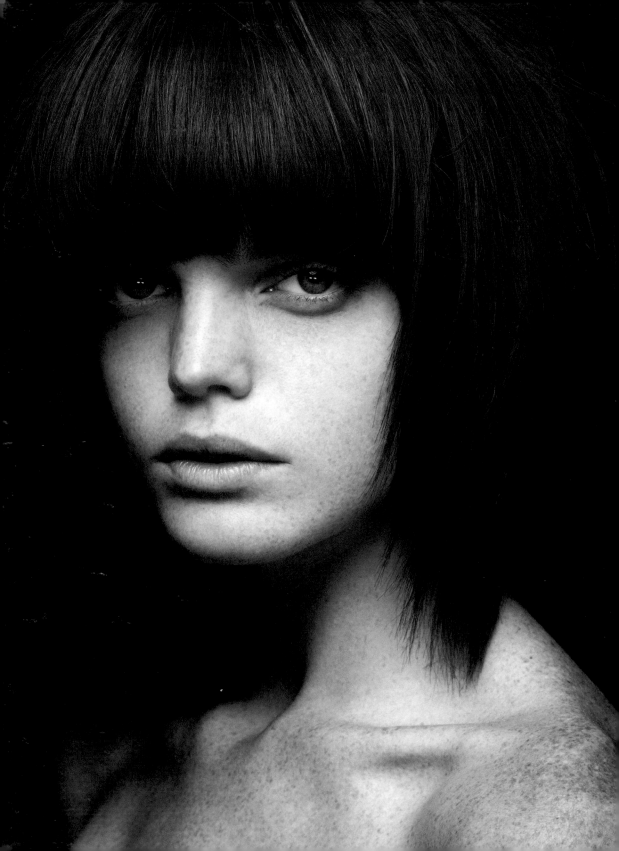

antique gold eyes

1 Clean up the brows. Prep the eye with foundation, but no powder. (You don't powder because you are applying the pigment with a wet brush, and powder will only make the pigment coagulate). Using a medium brush, apply an antique gold shadow to the entire lid.

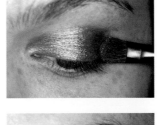

2 Continue the same gold pigment to the inner corner of the eye. Then apply an intense gold eyeliner to the inner rim and along the top eyelash line.

TIP

This is not the easiest of looks to achieve, so give yourself plenty of time to practise before you try it for an evening out. These eyes must be finished off with beautifully defined brows, otherwise the look doesn't seem finished.

3 Using a wet thin brush, apply a thin layer of cream blue-black pigment by drawing a diagonal line from the inner corner of the eye to the brow. The line should cut through the brow bone.

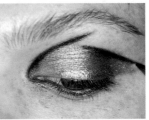

4 Using an angled brush, apply the blue-black pigment to the crease of the eye, following your natural socket line, beginning at the top and working downwards in a straight line. The line should end in line with the end of your brow. A steady hand is essential!

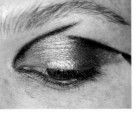

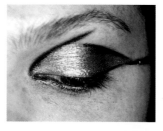

5 Extend the antique gold eye shadow into a triangular shape, then apply a very fine deep-blue eyeliner along the outer top lash line, and extend it out slightly.

LASHES USED

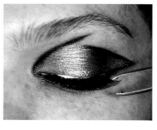

6 Curl lashes and apply a full set of false lashes. Notice I have applied a light-feathery lash as opposed to a heavy lash.

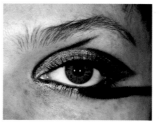

7 Apply black mascara to both the real and fake lashes to give a thicker effect. Make it slightly clumpy if you wish. This look is great for light-coloured lashes. Apply a gel blue-black eyeliner along the top lash line.

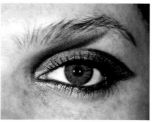

8 To soften the black line that extends from the inner corner to the brow bone, use a soft black eye shadow and lightly blend over it.

MODEL: ADA - CHIC MODELS • STYLING: JENNIFER SMIT - DLM

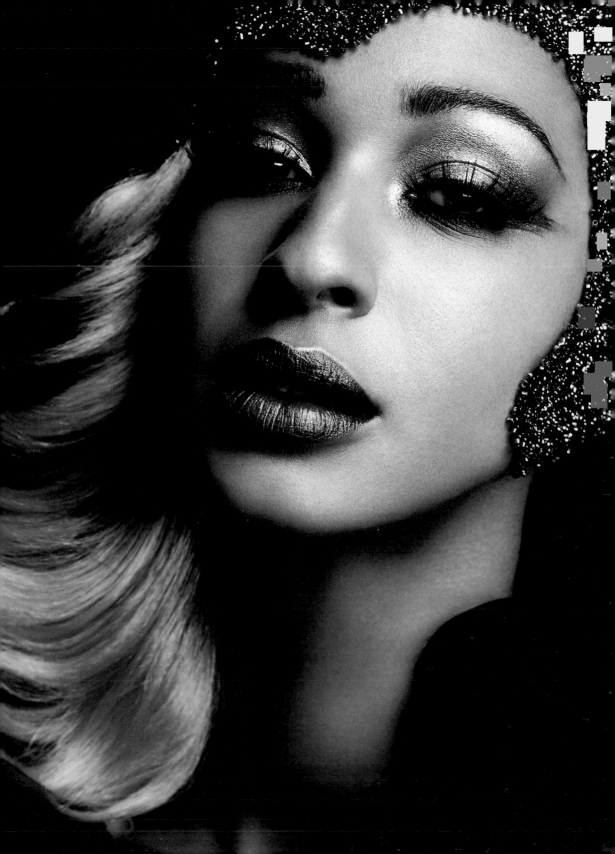

diva eyes

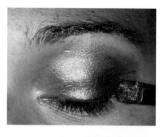

1 Prep the eye but don't powder. Wet your brush and apply a rose-gold pigment over the whole lid. Then apply a strong copper pigment over the lid but not as high as the first colour. This will blend the two colours beautifully. Don't look up for 1 minute to avoid creasing.

TIP
This look requires well-defined brows. You should clean up your brows before you prep your eyes.

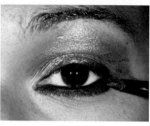

2 Apply a creamy black eyeliner to the inner lash rim and along one-third of the top lash line. Make sure this is smudged into the lash line, so there are no skin-coloured gaps along the lower lash line. It may look heavy at this stage, but you need this depth to create the eye shape.

3 Using a wet brush, apply black pigment to the outer corner of the eye and smudge. This creates depth and drama, and is great for small or closely set eyes.

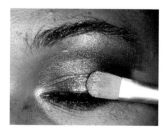

4 Apply an antique gold shadow heavily to the inner corner V of the eye, and smack bang in the middle of the eyelid. Also apply on the brow bone just under the eyebrow.

5 Define the brows. Curl the lashes and apply plenty of black mascara to the top and bottom lashes. Use a very strong false lash with eyelash glue.

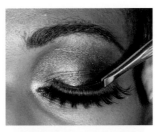

6 Apply lip balm to moisturise your lips and act as a base. Then apply pigment over the entire lips. Note that I'm using a metallic pigment as a lipstick. This is a good way to get strong lips, as most lipsticks will not give you this intensity.

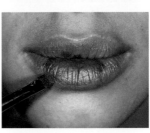

TIP
I am using black eyelash glue here to apply the false lashes. You can use white glue, but you may need a fair amount so it may take a while to dry.

7 Take the same antique gold used on the eye, and apply to the cupid's bow of the lips, and the middle of the bottom lip. I rarely recommend that women apply makeup using cotton buds, but they are perfect for applying the gold to the middle of the bottom lip.

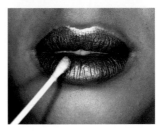

LASHES USED

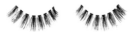

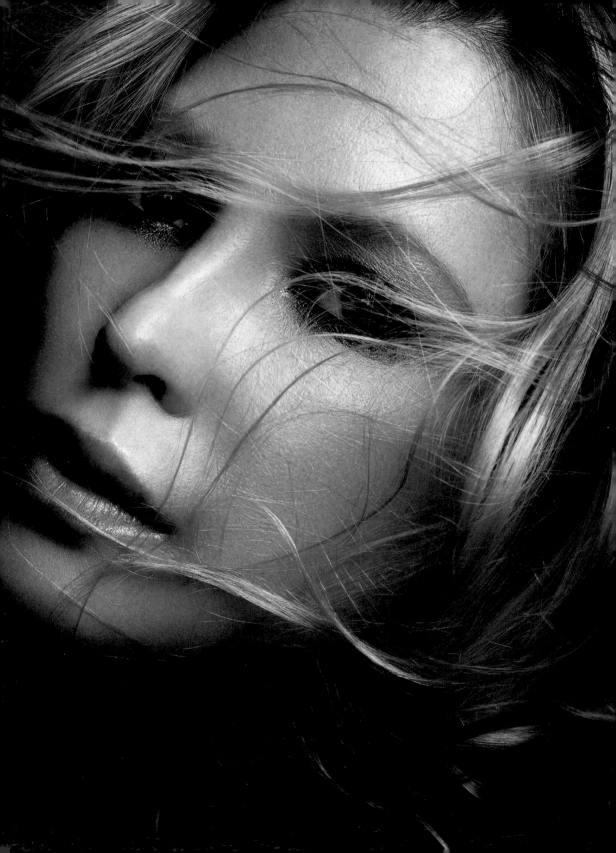

sensual eyes

1 Prep your eye then, using a medium brush, apply a golden copper pigment under the eye. Note that it's a few millimetres wide so that when you apply the darker shade it has something to blend out to.

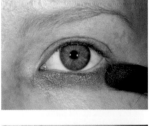

2 Apply the same pigment around the entire eye, carrying it up to the brow. Then apply a chocolate-brown metallic pencil to the inner rim of the eye (a matt brown pencil is also a great option).

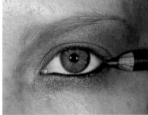

3 Using a thin brush, apply a dark mahogany brown to the upper lid, concentrating along the lash line. Note the shape is straight across the lid, not rounded. Apply this under the eye as well, intensifying it near the outer edge.

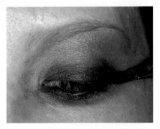

4 Finish by applying a black pigment around the eye, close to the lash line. Then add mascara to the top and bottom lashes.

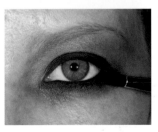

jewelled eyes

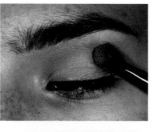

1 Prep the eyelid by making sure it is powdered well. Using a large brush, apply a light wash of soft coral eye shadow along the eye socket, blending up to the brow bone.

TIPS

This look is recommended for light olive to darker-toned skin.

This makeup looks best with strong top false lashes: it frames the eye.

For a cat-like eye effect, add mascara to the top lash line only. Only use black. Then finish off by using a soft gold highlighter under the brow.

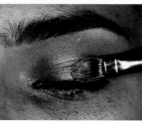

2 Using a large brush, cover the whole eyelid with an intense violet pigment, stopping just under the brow bone. Don't worry at this point about fallout— you can clean it up later. You can wet the brush to intensify the colour quickly.

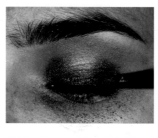

3 Using a smaller brush, intensify the lash line by applying a deeper shade of purple along the upper eyelid. You can also use a deep violet pencil or cream eyeliner to do this.

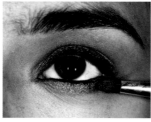

4 Clean up the drops of shadow that have fallen under the eye. Lightly base and powder under the eye (using a light dust of translucent powder for blending purposes). Then finish by applying an aqua-green pencil to the inner eye rim and shadow to the lower lash line, then mascara to the top and bottom lashes.

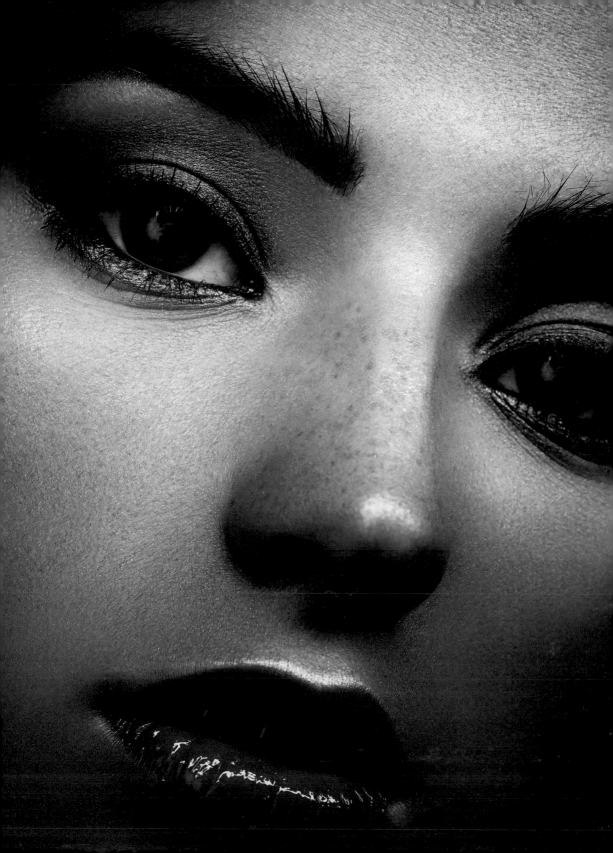

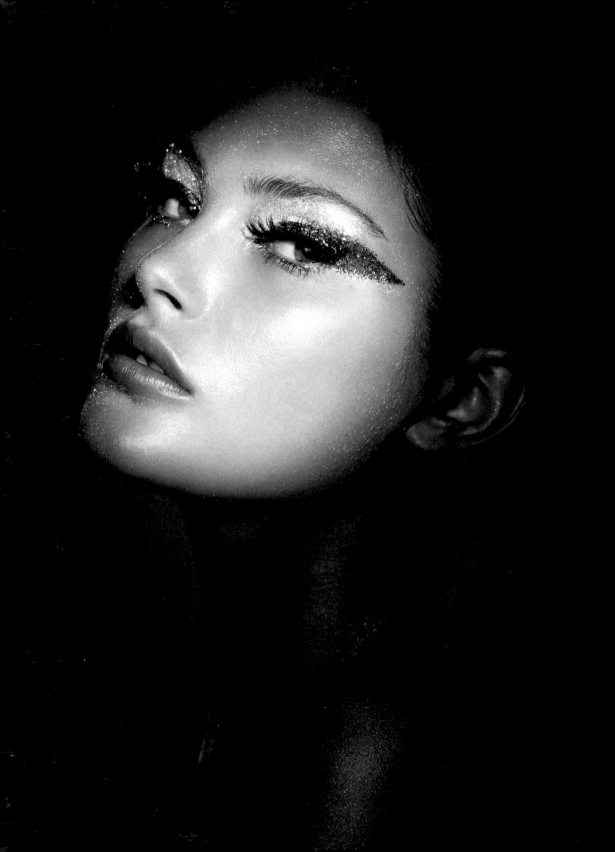

cleopatra eyes

1 Apply powder to all the places around the eye where the glitter is *not* meant to go: the brow bone, inner eye rim, beneath the eye and so on.

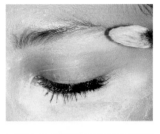

2 Paint eyelash glue on the eyelid. Only use a brush that you don't mind waving goodbye to. Wait until the glue is sticky and tacky before you apply the glitter, and only do one eye at a time, as getting glue in the eye can be very dangerous.

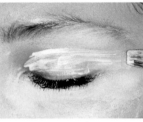

TIPS

Remember, only put eyelash glue where you want the glitter eye shadow to go.

I've finished off the look by dusting Catherine's skin with silver shimmer powder.

3 Using a medium brush, apply the charcoal or gunmetal-grey glitter evenly over the glue. Use a small hairdryer to blow off unwanted glitter.

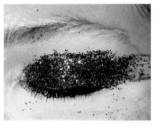

LASHES USED

4 Use masking tape to gently remove unwanted glitter remnants. Then use a cotton pad with Sorbolene cream to clean up under the eye. Gently wipe off any excess powder, and finish with foundation and mascara.

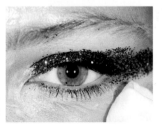

MODEL: SAM BLADES - CHIC MODELS • HAIR: MURIEL VANCAUWEN
• STYLING: JENNIFER SMIT - DLM • DRESS: AKIRA

lilac eyes

1 Using a medium brush, apply a soft wash of lavender to the eyelid, then add a little bit of white wash to the centre of the eyelid.

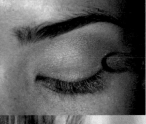

2 Starting from the inner eye socket, just under the brow bone, apply navy-black eye shadow in a fine line following the arch of the eyelid.

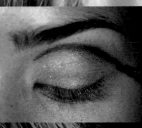

3 Clean up the fallout from the liner on the upper lid, by using a small brush with lavender eye shadow to blend.

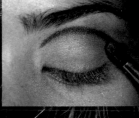

4 Comb brows. Wet your brush and apply a white frost pigment. Make sure the colour is translucent, to allow the original lavender colour to show through. Also apply heavily to the inner corner of the eye. Curl lashes and apply plenty of black mascara to the top lashes only.

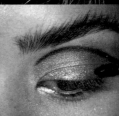

metallic eyes

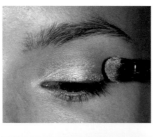

1 Prep the eyes but don't powder. Using a wet medium brush, apply a wash of metallic silver pigment to the whole eyelid. Make sure the application is quite fine, otherwise it will crack with time.

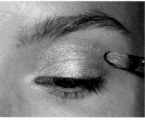

2 Wet the brush again, then apply a diamond dust (or paler shade of silver) to blend the colour higher to just under the brow bone. Also apply an extra amount to the middle of the eyelid. This gives a beautiful highlight.

LASHES USED

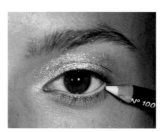

3 Apply an eggshell-white pencil to the inner rim of the eye. Remember, this will fade so you will need to reapply it.

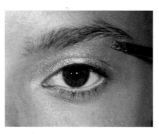

4 Apply a very intense diamond dust all over the eyelid and under the brows. Don't do this on eyes that are a bit puffy, as it will accentuate that puffiness. Finish by applying mascara to your top lashes and then applying fine false lashes.

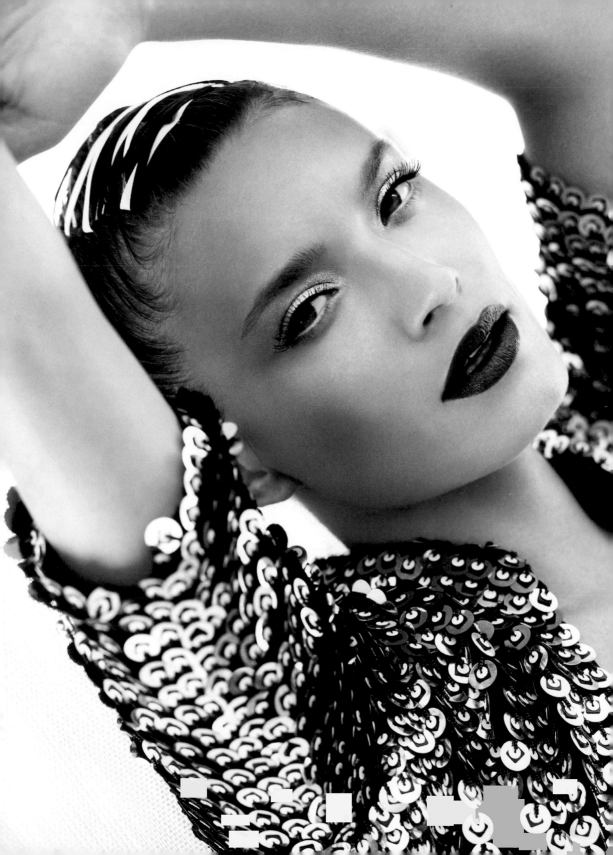

classic eyes

1 Prep the eyes and powder well. Using a large brush, apply a nude matt eye shadow to the whole eyelid.

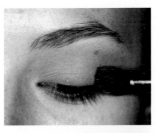

2 Using a thin brush, apply a taupe/oyster-grey shadow to the entire eyelid, and along the bottom lash line.

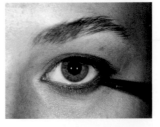

3 Apply a black eyeliner pencil to the inner rim of the eye. Apply the eyeliner heavier in the outer corner V of the eye—you can use a brush as shown.

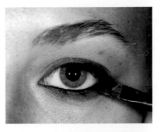

4 Curl lashes, then apply plenty of black mascara to both the top and bottom lashes.

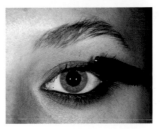

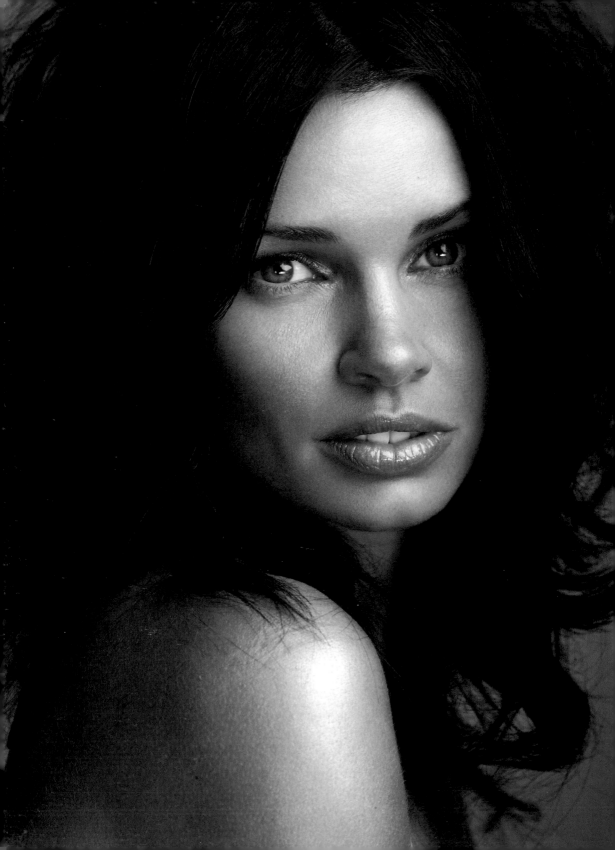

natural eyes

1 Prep the skin but don't powder. Use foundation mixed with illuminiser to give the skin a glowing finish. Then apply a soft gold glitter pigment all over the eyelid (don't go to the brow bone). This gives the illusion of dewy eyes.

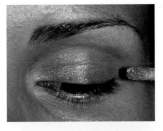

2 With the eyes open, apply an intense amount of glitter to the inner corner. Glitter gels are much better than loose glitter, as they don't get into the eye.

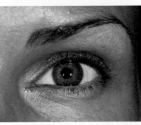

TIP
You don't need to prep the eye with powder for this look. If you need to, you can apply foundation to the eye, but it's not necessary.

3 Clean up and define the brows. Apply a thin coat of black mascara to the top lashes only. Comb it through when the lashes are still wet to prevent clumping.

4 Apply single false lashes to the outside of the top lashes. Finish by applying a cheek stain, and a pinky-peach gloss to the lips.

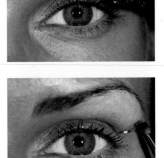

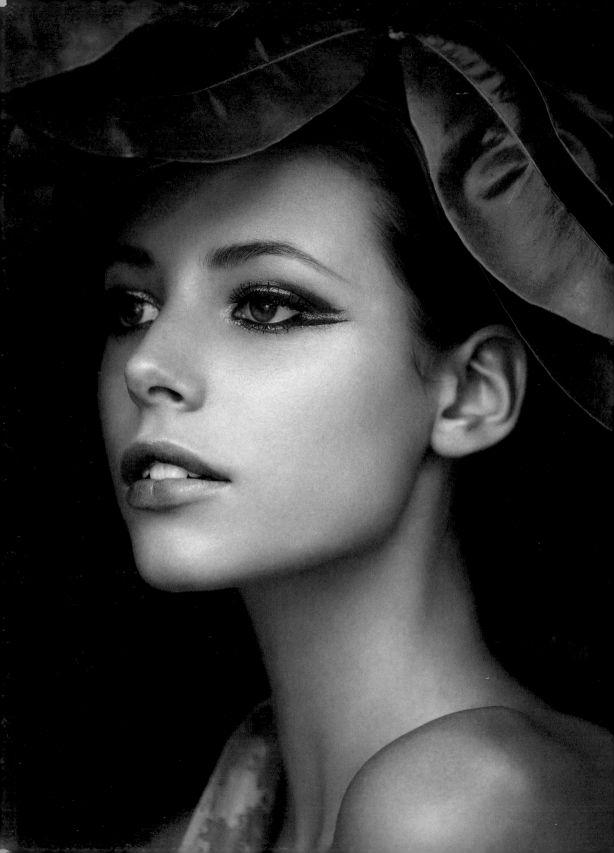

grecian eyes

1 Prep the eyes. Apply black eyeliner heavily to the inner rim of the eye, allowing it to thicken and drop a little as you extend it to the outer corner (as shown). Then, using a small brush, smudge the line and extend out on a slightly upward angle.

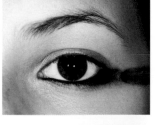

2 Dip a wet thin brush in copper pigment, then apply heavily to the under-lid as shown, keeping it close to the lash line, and stopping two-thirds of the way along.

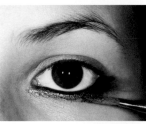

TIPS

The eye shadow should not go above the brow bone for this look.

This is not recommended for small eyes.

3 Wet your brush again, dip it in copper pigment and apply all over the eyelid. Wait for it to dry before you look straight ahead. If you don't want this intensity, you can apply a similar colour in a dry eye shadow.

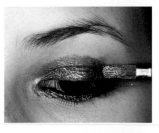

4 Apply black kohl pencil heavily to the outer corner of the eye. Let it sit a minute to allow your skin to heat it up; this makes it much easier to blend.

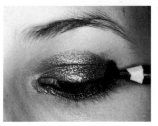

TIPS

If you wish, you can use another colour (instead of the copper) to cut the black in half.

This look is brilliant for rounded or bulging eyes, as the winged effect of the false eyelashes reshapes the eyes.

Be gentle when applying mascara over a false lash; if you use too much pressure, it will rip off. Make sure mascara is the very last thing you do, as having drops of pigment along the lash line can make the eye look dirty and unfinished.

LASHES USED

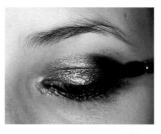

5 Dip a wet brush in black eye shadow, and blend into a V shape (as shown). Yes, this may be difficult, so you will need to practise. This blending is essential as you need to soften the edge. If you're struggling, dip a clean brush in translucent powder to blend the black.

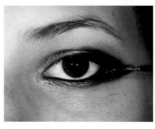

6 Using an eyeliner brush, apply copper pigment to the outer corner of the eye. The idea is to split the black shadow into two lines, as this is a very effective technique, and was used a lot in the 1960s (remember Twiggy?).

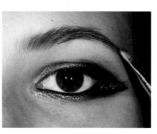

7 Using a brush, define your eyebrows with a soft eye shadow that is the same colour as your brow hair.

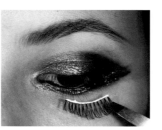

8 Curl lashes, then apply a full set of false lashes that have been cut to create a winged effect. Use eyelash glue to attach the lashes. Wait for it to to thicken before applying. Wait 5 minutes then apply black mascara to the top and bottom lashes.

acknowledgements

I would like to say a huge thankyou to all those who helped make this book possible:

Alethea Gold, without whom none of this would be possible; Richard Sharah, my mentor and the greatest makeup artist that ever lived; Jenny Hayes and Dotti.

Dolores Lavin - DLM, Ben Croft, Grace Testa - Studio Twenty4, Bronwyn Fraser (www.styleestablishment.com.au), Scott - ACMUSE, Maria - Makeup Store, Jo - MAC and Jodi Gardner.

Steven Chee, Katie Nolan, Dan Nadel, Kate Ursi and Matt.

My literary agents Mark Byrne and Lisa Hanrahan, and my publisher Jude McGee and editor Alexandra Nahlous.

My assistants Victoria Baron, Rachel Brook, Nicole Rossetto, Jane Drew, Ana Slavka, Sandra Cook, Nikki Halsted, Giorgi Ciot, Mandi Levanah - DLM, Martin Bray - The Artist Group and Cassie Sobel and the students of Cameron Jane Makeup School.

Special thanks for the expert advice of Dr Van Park B.Sc. (Med). M.B.B.S., F.R.A.C.G.P. and Dr Peter L. Dixon M.B.B.S. F.R.A.C.S.

Stylists: Jennifer Smit - DLM, Michael Azzollini, Richard Milvain and Wil Ariyamethe - DLM.

Hair: Brad Ballard, Dario Cotroneo using GHD, Julianne McGuigan - DLM, Karen Hopwood - DLM, Lores Giglio - DLM, Michael Brennan - The Artist Group, Muriel Vancauwen RP Represents www.rprepresents.com and Raymond Robinson - DLM.

Illustrators: Nigel Stanislaus and Dennis White.

Models: Abbey - Bella Model Management & Ford Models, New York, Ada - Chic Models, Alice - Chic Models, Annika - Chic Models, Bianca - Chic Models, Camille Piazza - Chic Models, Cassie - Chic Models, Catherine McNeil - Chic Models, Cheyenne Tozzi - Priscillas Model Management, Emma Booth - William Morris, Eunice Ward - Chadwick, Felicity King - Vivien's, Florence - Chic Models, Gemma Poole - Vivien's, Gemma Stooke - Priscillas Model Management, Jamie Moore - Scoop Management, Jodi Gardner - Chic Models, Kate Alstergren - Mark Byrne Management, Katie Lange - Chadwick, Kieta - Chic Models, Kirstie Penn - Chic Models, Kristine Duran - Chic Models, Lara Bingle, Lizzy B - Chic Models, Lucy Bayet - Chadwick, Michelle Leslie, Miranda Kerr - Chic Models, Olivia Dunnfrost - Chadwick, Renee Mansbridge - Chic Models, Sam Blades - Chic Models, Sarah Grant - Mark Byrne Management, Sonya Kukainis - Vivien's, Stephanie Carta - Chic Models, Tottie Goldsmith, Valerija - Chic Models, Ursula Hufnagl, Dr Van Park and Xiya Xu - Vivien's.

And finally, thank you to Dov for all the terrific catering, Echelon Studios, Justin Braitling - Location House, David and Melinda Itzkowic - Location House, Kellie Tissear, Francis Callanan, Jeremy Southern and John Williams.

index